1 MONTH OF
FREE
READING

at

www.ForgottenBooks.com

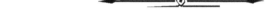

By purchasing this book you are eligible for one month membership to ForgottenBooks.com, giving you unlimited access to our entire collection of over 700,000 titles via our web site and mobile apps.

To claim your free month visit:

www.forgottenbooks.com/free435796

ISBN 978-0-483-58105-0
PIBN 10435796

DISSERTATION

ON

GOUT;

EXHIBITING

A NEW VIEW OF THE ORIGIN, NATURE, CAUSE, CURE, AND
PREVENTION,

OF THAT

𝕬fflicting 𝕯isease;

ILLUSTRATED AND CONFIRMED BY

A VARIETY OF ORIGINAL AND COMMUNICATED CASES.

BY ROBERT KINGLAKE, M. D.

Member of the Royal Medical Society of Edinburgh, of the Physical
Society of Gottingen, &c. &c. and Physician at Taunton.

Medicina in philosophia, non fundata, res infirma est.—BACON.

LONDON;

PRINTED FOR JOHN MURRAY, NO. 32, FLEET STREET;
BELL AND BRADFUTE, EDINBURGH; AND GILBERT
AND HODGES, DUBLIN.

1804.

S. GOSNELL, Printer, Little Queen Street, Holborn.

THE DUKE OF PORTLAND.

MY LORD DUKE,

THE honour which your Grace has conferred on me, in liberally permitting this new work on Gout to be addressed to your notice, is enhanced by the prospect of its affording your Grace that lively interest, which you must necessarily feel in every attempt to cure a disease, which has afflicted with deplorable inveteracy your illustrious ancestors, and from the severity of which your own health has not been exempted.

If the mode of treatment recommended in this performance should be earlier adopted

by

by the community in general, and by the
higher classes of society in particular, from
your Grace's attention being especially invited to it, than if its publication were less
auspiciously distinguished, my object in
this Dedication will be accomplished; and
the event promises to be too gratifying to
your Grace's science and benevolence, for
you ever to regret having granted the indulgence.

It cannot be presumed that your Grace's
ideas on the subject of Gout, should have
been wholly unclouded by the prevailing
medical and popular prejudices, on the nature and tendency of that disease; but it
may be confidently expected, that your
intelligent readiness to be convinced, by
competent testimony, will secure to this production your careful perusal, and at least,
an admission of the facts it contains.

Increasing

Increasing familiarity with the proposed remedy, accumulating evidence of its superior efficacy, and your Grace's deep personal stake in a plan that professes always promptly to alleviate, and in general radically to cure Gout, must ultimately prove, in your Grace's correct judgment, duly persuasive.

I have the honour to be,

MY LORD DUKE,

With profound respect,

Your Grace's

Much obliged and most obedient servant,

ROBERT KINGLAKE.

Taunton,
July 5th, 1804.

PREFACE.

I⊤ may be proper to apprise the reader, that the ensuing pages offer a new view of the nature and cure of gouty affection.

A disease, which has hitherto. baffled every curative effort of medical art, and has universally been deemed either *salutary* or *incurable*, cannot be affirmed to be an ailment equally *noxious* and *curable*, without alarming prevailing prejudices, and provoking opposition.

Whatever obloquy may befall my endeavour to correct the errors of science, and of vulgar adoption, on this subject, it will not repress my ardour for establishing the truth of *positions* so important, as that Gout differs in no essential circumstance from common inflammation; that it is not a constitutional, but merely a local affec-

tion;

tion; that its genuine seat is exclusively in the ligamentous and tendinous structure; that its attack is never salutary; that it should neither be encouraged nor protracted; and that, if seasonably and appropriately treated, it is as easily remediable as inflammatory excitement on the muscular, cuticular, or any other description of organic texture.

The subject is here freely discussed, independently of either academic or individual authority; it is therefore expected, that the doctrine advanced will find no quarter where vulnerable, nor that it can possibly resist the torrent of assailment, which its originality challenges, but by its own intrinsic correctness.

If the shafts of criticism should be pointed with convincing argument, they may usefully reach the mark of truth; but if barbed with invective or contumely, they may inflict illiberal reproach, but will want the peculiar force of persuasive candour.

The

The treatment here proposed for Gout, was deduced from theory: the effects of the treatment confirm at least the practical value of that theory, if not its philosophical justness.

Whatever, therefore, may be the fate of my reasoning in public estimation, the facts which have resulted from it will, in permanency, class with the physical elements of nature, will endure as long as the present economy of the universe, and when the author and his commentators shall have immemorially passed away, in the mighty wreck of decomposing substances!

" Quantacunque fuerint aliorum conamina, semper existimavi mihi vitalis auræ usum frustra datum fore, nisi et ipse, in hoc studio versatus, symbolum aliquod, utcunque exiguum, in commune medicinæ ærarium contribuerem."— SYDENHAM.

THE AUTHOR.

Taunton,
July 5th, 1804.

CONTENTS.

SECTION I.

Origin of Gout.

SECTION II.

Nature and Constitution of Gout.

SECTION III.

Remote and proximate Cause of Gout.

SECTION IV.

Cure of Gout.

SECTION V.

Prevention of Gout.

SECTION VI.

Recapitulation.

APPENDIX.

EXPLANATIONS.

To prevent any obscurity which may arise to the general or unprofessional reader, from the few technical terms occurring in this Dissertation, the subsequent definitions are alphabetically prefixed.

Articular—Appertaining to a joint.

Associative—Synonymous with Sympathetic, but a more descriptive term of the manner in which the motive connexion of parts obtains.

Bronchial—Relating to the air-vessels of the lungs, or to the branches of the windpipe.

Cartilaginous—Relating to the soft polished substances, with which the extremities of bones, forming the joints, are tipped or surmounted.

Dyspeptic—Relating to difficult digestion.

Excitability—Synonymous with Irritability, but more literally expressive of the innate liability to be acted on, or excited by stimulant powers.

Excretion—The removal of the fluids, secreted or separated from the mass of blood, out of the body.

Fascial

Fascial—Relating to an expansion of a dense strong texture, called tendinous, over the more active muscles, to limit and sustain their exertion.

Hepatic—Relating to the liver.

Humoral—Referring to humours or vitiated fluids, erroneously supposed to be generated in the body, to circulate with the blood, and to occasion diseases, only curable by either expelling them to the skin, or rejecting them by some excreting outlet.

Ligament, or *Ligamentous Structure*—Is a compact, dense, bloodless texture, both connecting and investing the heads or portions of bones forming the joints.

Locomotive—Relating to a power of moving from one place to another, as possessed by animal life, in contradistinction to that of vegetable.

Osseous—Of the nature of bone.

Pathological—Relating to the nature and doctrine of diseases.

Periosteal—Appertaining to the membrane, or covering which immediately invests the bones of the animal body.

Peristaltic—Belonging to the peculiar motions of the bowels, by which their feculent contents are protruded, and finally ejected.

Pneumonic—Relating to the lungs.

Secretion—Is a vascular action, or process, by which various kinds of fluids are formed and separated from the mass of blood, such as saliva, urine, bile, &c.

Stomachic—Relating to the stomach.

Tendon,

Tendon, or *Tendinous Structure*—-A dense, compact, strong substance, similar in texture to that of the ligament, or ligamentous structure, forming the extremities of muscles, and attached to the ligamentous and bony fabric of the joints, serving as a pulley or lever to the muscular action, in moving the joints.

Tracheal—Relating to the windpipe.

Visceral—Relating to the vital organs, such as the brain, heart, stomach, &c.

———————

The Reader is requested to correct the following Errata.

Page 72, line 21, *for* now, *read* new.
    76, —— 16, *for* determinal, *read* determinate.
    88, —— 15, *for* medical, *read* medicinal.
    173, —— 1, *erase the confused letters which stand for the third word, and substitute* immersion.
    178, —— 21, *after the word* two, *read* as a.
    193, —— 1, *after* permit, *read* me.

DISSERTATION,

&c.

SECTION I.

ORIGIN OF GOUT.

1. THE origin of gout must have been nearly coeval with that of human existence; since both the physical and moral causes, which give birth to it, must have occasionally prevailed in the earliest ages of mankind. The medical writings * indeed of remote antiquity have transmitted records of the gout being known as a familiar disease.

That this distemper should have occurred so early, rests on a law of the animal economy, which must always have subjected the human frame

* Those of Hippocrates, Aretæus, Galen, Alexander, &c.

to

to the operation of its efficient causes: but it is strikingly singular, that nearly the same opinion should have been entertained of its nature during so long a period.

2. To no other influence than that of humoral pathology could the inveteracy with which the gout has invariably preserved its reputation as a critical or curative malady have been owing.

The authority of this doctrine has proscribed, with peculiar strictness, all inquiry into the disease, which did not recognise its salutary tendency, as a leading and regulating principle in its examination and management.

When formality of science decrees, and popular assent adopts an incorrect notion of disease, more than common effort of intellect, and more than ordinary regard for independent reasoning, are necessary, freely to canvass its merits, and boldly to expose its errors.

The crapulous and highly distempered health of those who more particularly suffered from gout, speciously imposed a persuasion, that the local affection must have resulted from the disordered system, and that fatal dangers had been eluded

by

by so favourable a deposit of morbid influence. This opinion became current, was implicitly accredited, and solemnly sanctioned.

3. Protracted gout, whether acquired or hereditary, is foremost in the catalogue of evils that has arisen from adopted prejudices as to the nature and cure of disease. If freedom of inquiry, if independence of authority, and exclusive devotion to the evidence of facts be ever necessary, they are surely so in contemplating the conditions of health and disease.

Can a liberal regard for the advancement of medical science endure the impediments which are thrown in the way of improvement, by arrogant opinions of competent proficiency having been made in speculations at once replete with interest and doubt ? Is the habit of an opinion to ensure its continuance in defiance of every opportunity, of every occasion for its correction ?

Medical prejudices have and will exist, but they neither have nor should justify an abject surrender of inquisitorial right.

Had unfounded doctrines of diseases met early and unremitted opposition, errors would not

have

have been privileged by custom ; but an emulous spirit of inquiry would have progressively extended the bounds of real intelligence.

A disposition to adopt, rather than to scrutinize, has had the pernicious influence of lulling every desire for rational research into a lethargic indifference for improvement ; and induced an indolent satisfaction with what exists, rather than a thoughtful endeavour to elucidate and explain difficulties.

4. The extreme tardiness, the reluctant caution, indeed, with which the errors of humoral pathology have given way to a more correct and enlightened view of disease, seems to have reserved gout as an exception to its illustrative influence.

The plague, every variety of putrid fever, the exanthematous, or eruptive affections, more particularly the small-pox and measles, though for ages bound in the fetters of erroneous, of unyielding prejudices, at length escaped the deadly trammels by the irresistible force of common sense, assisted by accidental instruction.

Although

. Although the authority of established doctrine licensed the pursuit of a hurtful mode of treatment, and offered an admissible vindication for its consequences, yet it has not been wholly lost to observation, that occasionally the reverse of the plan of cure espoused and prosecuted, was signally successful.

If the efforts of febrile delirium accidentally liberated the burning patient from his confinement, by enabling him to escape from his fiery durance, and, without clothing, to expose himself to cold air; or, more extensively impelled by sensation, to precipitate himself into cold water; prompt and radical relief was afforded, to the utter astonishment and confusion of the curative attempts which had been founded on the efficacy of accumulated heat.

Reiterated proof of the salutary influence of reduced temperature, in variolous and typhous affections, was thus casually furnished, before an improved view of the nature of those diseases justified it by principle, and recommended it to general adoption.

If the principle could be once admitted, that diseases characterized by extreme heat might be

B 3   saf y

safely and advantageously combated by reduced
temperature, and that by such treatment their
malignant nature and progress might be repressed, without incurring any mischief from
repulsion, it discovers a singular neglect of analogical reasoning not to have applied it to the
case of acute gout, in which the criteria of inflammation, and the distempered heat by which
it is induced, were most glaring.

It is true, gouty affection is more distinguished
as a local disease than any other form of either
febrile or inflammatory disorder, and the subjects
of it have been in general but too conscious of
irregularities in mode of living, that are sufficient
to induce constitutional malady. This persuasion has kept gout within the pale of humoral
pathology, and obstinately barricaded it with the
fostering ordinances of flannel, patience, and
sedulous stimulation.

That error should have existed, necessarily results from inexperience; but that it should inveterately resist the clear evidence of close analogy,
can only be ascribed to the senseless inflexibility
of habitual prejudice. Delay of improvement
finds some remuneration in its ultimate maturity.
It renders conviction more decisive, and affords
an

an instructive example of the delusion into which the judgment has been betrayed, either by the sophistry of reasoning, or the stupid habit of unintelligent adoption.

If it should appear, that the nature of gout has for ages been involved in obscurity, by gratuitous reasoning concerning it, and that its prevailing mode of treatment has protracted its fits, and unnecessarily extended its various evils to the constitution, it must be admitted on fair analogy, that other diseases supposed to be of a kindred nature, in depurating the system, and locally depositing morbid influence, should lose all claim to confidence for remedial agency, and be consigned to their just station in the rank of positive ailments, demanding the best and earliest effort of medical skill to check their progress, and annul their existence.

SECTION

SECTION II.

NATURE AND CONSTITUTION OF GOUT.

1. GOUT is a greater or less degree of inflammatory affection of the ligaments and tendons, induced by distempered excitability of those parts from various causes.

Its true nature consists of active inflammation, assuming every diversity which constitutional and temperamental conditions of life and health may impart to it; but in all cases, it inflicts on the affected parts, the morbid changes characteristic of inflammatory violence.

It is an erroneous notion, that it may be constituted by transient excitement, without the more stationed features of inflammation. This is transient irritation only, and wants the essential and more durable circumstances of definite gout.

Were all pains darting through the joints to be deemed gouty, the appellation would assume the general latitude assigned to indiscriminate
                                              irritation,

irritation, and would distinguish with no precision the well-marked form of disease termed
gout.

The sentient principle of life is indeed often
tortured in parts, without inducing that vascular
afflux of fluids, distention, and excitement,
which are necessary to constitute gouty, in common with every other description of inflammation. On those occasions, the pain proceeds
from distempered sensibility, insulated, and concentrated, on nervous structure. Gouty irritation has a different seat, and an unrestrained
diffusion.

2. Idiopathic, or true gout, or rather that
inflammatory affection of the joints, which popular consent has denoted by that name, has its
station exclusively in the ligamentous and tendinous structure. The dense compactness of this
fabric gives to its nervous, vascular, and cellular
substances, sentient, irritative, and resisting
powers, peculiarly adapted to induce the painful
conflict sustained, when, from any cause, these
parts are subjected to inflammatory violence.
Strong derivant excitement, impulsive afflux of
fluids, and unyielding contractility of vessel, are
sufficient

sufficient to furnish the most distressful phenomena of gout.

If this disease, then, has for its seat organic texture, that imparts to it a specific modification, it is obvious that a different arrangement of parts must be incapable of affording precisely similar effects; and that consequently where this structure does not present, whatever be the morbid excitement, the formality of gout cannot be strictly recognised.

3. Different degrees of inflammatory affection of the ligaments and tendons have been erroneously supposed to be essentially distinct diseases, and have accordingly received such respective denominations, as have been held to be appropriate: thus an inflammation on those parts, arising from general causes, is at one time distinguished by the term rheumatism; at another, when the inflammatory irritation has resulted from external violence, particularly that of extension, it is named sprain. It will require no extraordinary skill in independent thinking, to perceive the perfect identity of these several nominal states of inflammation, and to refuse assent to the prevailing prejudice, that they are essentially different.

By

By a law of physical necessity, it must be admitted, that causes acting in similar circumstances, must produce similar effects; and an established rule of true philosophising forbids a reference to superfluous agency in explanation of efficient power *. An active inflammation of the ligamentous and tendinous structure presents an example of the constituent parts suffering from the excitement of increased motion and tension. The degree of the affection will be proportioned to the violence of the impressing cause, and the greater or less irritable state of the parts subjected to the disease; but these different degrees of excitement create no real difference in the quality of the effect, however it may have been induced.

If the stomach be solicited to a rejection of its contents, by virtue of ipecacuanha at one time, and by tartarised antimony at another, in both cases the effect is vomiting; and, however it may differ in degree, the physical conditions in the operation are identically the same.

Why then, in servile conformity to unmeaning custom, shall medical language authorize a dis-

* See Newton's Principia, Rules 1st and 2d.

tinction.

tinction without a difference, in variously denominating the same affection, gouty, rheumatic,
and ligamentous or tendinous inflammation ?

The fundamental identity of these ideally different inflammations, cannot be questioned from
the external differences which accidentally diver-
sify the form of the effect.

Rheumatic inflammation, in the received opinion of its nature, denotes a condition of ligamentous, and tendinous irritation, less exclusively
confined to these parts, than occurs in that form
of affection which is termed gout. In the rheumatic aspect of the disease the inflammation
extends farther, and more rapidly to the muscular
fabric, and generates more remote, and transient
sympathies.

In consequence of this diffused and incessantly
renewing irritation on joints, with which the
motive influence of associated excitability has
been more particularly established, the system
at large participates more constantly in the
morbid irritation, and exhibits, in common
estimation, a farther feature of dissimilitude to
gout.

It

It is much easier to theorize and fabricate distinct doctrines on the diversified appearances of disease, than to withdraw the veil of prejudice that prevents a correct generalization of them. It is not difficult to affirm, that an inflammatory affection of a joint may at one time be limited to the ligamentous and tendinous parts; and that, at another, it may be indefinitely extended either over the aponeurotic expansion, or sheath of the adjoining muscles, or to the muscular fabric itself; but does it satisfactorily follow, that there is any radical difference in the origin and nature of these unequally extended affections; and that the one should be designated by the term gout, the other by that of rheumatism?

Were these external lines of demarcation, indeed, uniformly steady, a formal distinction in the disease might be indulged; but this not being the case, and there being no reason why the more confined and extensive irritations should not be considered (as they in fact really are) interchangeable conditions of the same affection, governed by accidental circumstances, it would be uselessly multiplying names to allow them distinct appellations.

Experience

Experience bears ample testimony to the extreme difficulty of applying the prevailing ground
of distinction between gout and rheumatism.
Medical practitioners are often inextricably per-
plexed with the diagnostic phantom of gout and
rheumatism.   In consultation it becomes a subject of awful discussion.   The irascible and
bigotted are apt to dissent violently, sometimes
indeed opprobriously ; the demure more gravely;
whilst the polite conformist compromises the difficulty, by denominating it rheumatic gout.
Such puerilities surely are unworthy of medical
science, and should not be tolerated in a philosophical age.

The inflammation induced on the ligaments
and tendons by external violence, and which
is significantly termed sprain, discovers as strong
an identity with gouty irritation, as occurs in
rheumatic affection.   The same parts are subjected to inflammatory excitement, and the same
effects are consequently manifested.   Exquisite
pain, immobility of the affected joint, efflorescence, shining tumefaction, associative affection of other joints, and more or less of systematic irritation, at once characterize ligamentous
and tendinous extension, called sprain, and
                                        present

present an imposing catalogue of either gouty or rheumatic symptoms.

Without creating any real difference in the nature of the disease, the healthy excitability of the ligaments and tendons, may render the accidental irritation from extension or sprain, less afflicting, and more easily removeable, than when these parts, from having been subjected to repeated inflammatory attacks, have probably suffered in organic structure, and have certainly acquired a distempered susceptibility for morbid impression.

Repeated sprains tend to impair the organic tone, and vitiate the excitability of the affected parts, in the same manner as frequently renewed and protracted attacks of gout. Nor does the analogical influence cease here, but is even similarly extended, by associative or sympathetic motion, to the ligamentous and tendinous structure of other joints.

It is a law in the organic movements of the animal economy, not only that similar structure necessarily evolves similar action, but that the healthy, as well as distempered conditions of that action, are also associatively bound in indis-

soluble

soluble participation.—Sprain, therefore, repeatedly occurring on the same ligaments and tendons, will at once render them additionally
liable to inflammatory extension from external
accident, and to gouty irritation from the usual
causes, with all its morbid sympathies with other
joints.

As in gouty inflammation, so that from sprain
has no tendency to suppurate; the density of the
parts affected, the want of capacious cellular
texture, and sufficient afflux of fluids, concur
to resist such a termination.

Ligamentous excitability, stimulated to the extent of inflammatory action, may assume different forms, but changes not its fundamental
nature. In the lumbago, or disease of the lumbar
vertebral ligaments, the sciatica or hip-gout, the
white swelling or ligamentous inflammation, and
thickening of the knee, and other joints, are
various examples of inflammatory excitement
of the same structure as that which is the seat
of gouty irritation; and these acknowledge no
other difference than what consists in degree
and situation.

4. It

4. It is much to be regretted that the local origin of gout should have been so generally overlooked, both in the medical and popular notion of the nature of the malady. It has been gratuitously supposed, that gout is always a constitutional disease, and that the external inflammatory affection only marks its critical deposit. This opinion is founded on a very superficial, or rather on no philosophical view whatever of the disease; it was imagined when the reveries of humoral pathology embarrassed medical speculations, and authorized doctrines strangely at variance with common sense.

In the humoral view of the cause of diseases, it has been uniformly taken for granted, that something offensive, a *materies morbi*, has disturbed the harmony of health, and that the native powers of life, impatient of the injury, expel the morbid matter on situations securely distant from the visceral regions of life. Consonantly to this principle, it is to the present day obstinately held, that the gout provokes a salutary struggle in the system for the final expulsion of the disease to the extremities.

In questioning the veracity of this doctrine, it must be demanded, what proof exists of morbid

c   matter

matter pervading the system in constitutional gout; and when imaginarily deposited, where, or in what manner, can its local establishment be recognised? Has even the most confident votary to the humoral doctrine of gout attempted to explain the possibility of such a matter as is generated by the morbid actions of the gouty part, ever circulating with the mass of fluids, meandering through the brain and heart, and mingling in the various secretions, without bearing with it, in every conceivable instance, the most agonising destruction of life? Can it, in the utmost licentiousness of imagination, be for a moment thought, that a vital part of the system could participate in generating a matter so highly stimulant, as violently to inflame and insufferably torture the ligamentous and tendinous structure on its first deposition? or, in defiance of the acknowledged law of organic susceptibility for impression, will it be said that an agent virulent enough to kindle the most painful inflammation on a joint, may arrive thither with impunity to the transmitting parts?

These and other difficulties needless to adduce, are insuperably in the way of admitting the existence of gouty matter in the system, previously to its external determination. Such an untenable view

view of disease as is here exhibited, nauseates the love of truth, and turns the attention to a more promising search after it.

The phenomena of gout, correctly contemplated, offer irresistible evidence in proof of its genuine nature and origin. It is invariably founded in different degrees of inflammatory action, and its specific character requires that either the ligamentous or tendinous structure should be the seat of the affection. In every case, therefore, it may be considered as of local origin, though producible by various constitutional states of excitability, as well as injury primarily befalling the affected parts.

It will be hereafter seen, that various causes connected with temperature, diet, and constitution, operating on systematic excitability, may, from accidental preponderance of motive susceptibility on the ligaments and tendons, finally exert a concentrated or inflammatory influence on those parts, and thus induce the formal character of local gout. It must not then be contended, that the gout constitutionally existed before its appearance on the affected parts, as that would involve the solecism of giving being to a nonentity.

Consti-

Constitutional gout would presuppose constitutional fabric of ligament and tendon, in a state of inflammatory action from excessive excitement. The physical conditions, or requisite structure, therefore, to give effect to what is strictly understood by gouty inflammation, can only be found in the joints. What is erroneously termed gout in the system, is no more than distempered excitability, whether occurring originally or symptomatically, which may be concentrated or determined on the articular fabric, where it may be considered as an aggravation of the disease, by increasing the previous degree of painful irritation, and in no instance to be remedial.

As rationally may an inflammation of the brain arising from dyspeptic irritation in the stomach, be considered as an eligible remedy, as that the exquisite pain attendant on inflamed ligaments and tendons should be held to operate beneficially to the general health.

Pain at once gives name and virulence to disease; and in proportion as aggrieved sensibility prevails, is the danger of the existing malady : it cannot therefore, consistently with any rational view of healing, or curative endeavour, be admitted, that gout, or an inflammation so horribly

3 painful

painful as that of the ligaments and tendons, can salutarily avail in either annulling or repressing any morbid commotion of the system. On the contrary, it will be found, that this commotion is merely a sympathetic extension of the pain of the affected parts, and is invariably proportioned, both in degree and inveteracy, to the violence and protraction of the local disease.

. The importance of assigning to gout its structural character and local position, derives additional weight from the consideration, that the prevailing practice of tolerating it as a critical deposit, exposes the temperament to the worst effects of associative irritation, obtaining fixed establishment, from the powerful influence of fostered habit.

5. The symptomatic irritation diffused throughout the system, as well as its preponderance on any particular organ, in painful gout, will be governed by associative influence, whether healthful or morbid.

However gout originates, whether from external violence, or a distempered state of the general excitability, determined to the ligamentous and tendinous parts, the effect on the system will be similar. A painful source of irritation will be-

come

come established on more or less of the joints, and be incessantly propagated to the system at large.

If any particular organ should be previously disturbed by any unhealthful conditions of its motive powers or excitability, on that part the gouty excitement is liable more particularly to be arrested, where it will endure with greater or less violence, as it may happen to be incessantly deriving its support from the gouty source, or become independent of its exciting cause.

The stomach, for example, during a paroxysm of gout, may have its excitability so painfully impressed by a sympathetic or associative extension of the stimulant influence of that malady, as to be rendered unequal, either to its digestive function, or to that of supporting a sort of regulating tone and energy for the salutarily motive relations of the system generally. In that case, an ailment at the stomach may continue to prevail after the extinction of gouty pain, owing to the deep impression made on its native powers, unlike the transient effect arising from the slighter influence of morbid sympathy.

The fatal tendency of pain, or distempered sensation, in the animal economy, has lost its just terrors,

terrors, in the chimerical notions entertained of the more destructive operation of morbific matter. To the former is tritely offered as a solacing explanation, that it is merely nervous, while the latter is sabled with the horrors of inducing invincible disease, and even death, if not seasonably expelled. This worse than gratuitous reasoning, this hackneyed nonsense, has led to much undue management of disease, and has too often ensured the destruction of life, under an anxious formality of affording it protection.

It is one of the most provident conditions of animal life, that morbid matter is not a transferable evil. The motive powers of organic structure effectually bar its diffusion in a material form. They are susceptible of being impressed by it, and morbidly agitated by its influence; but there the mischief stops; and previously to its farther propagation, or systematic dissemination, it must assume the motive form which vital action imparts to it.

In this state it acquires an identity with vital power, vitiating its excitability, and becoming subject to the same laws of motive diffusion.

As

As every description of morbid influence results from altered conditions of native power, an incessant effort will be making to reassume the salutary state, by the innate and habitual force of health. This natural provision for recovery should encourage an unyielding confidence in the general curability of diseases, and more particularly in that of the gout, which is evidently a removable state of disordered action, threatening only to become immovable by the prejudicial custom of tolerating and cherishing it with indefinite patience.

6. The local symptoms of gout are strictly those of active inflammation of the ligamentous and tendinous parts, which, from natural density of structure, are not immediately susceptible of a morbid degree of irritation and sentient commotion. The motive powers of these parts, therefore, are for some time previously to the accession of violent inflammation, acquiring distempered excitability, evinced in uneasy sensation, arising in the fabric of the affected ligaments and tendons sympathetically exciting contractile pain, more or less transient, on the neighbouring muscles : this effect occasionally ranges by associative influence, far from the affected joint, and is known by the term cramp, or spasm, which in

strictness

strictness is an irregularity in muscular contraction, both in force and time. If the constituent fibres of muscular structure do not act simultaneously and in natural direction, a conflict arises between the extending and contracting powers, and involves the affected parts in painful stiffness.

The comparatively unexcitable state of the ligamentous and tendonous structure is confined to the influence of first impression only; it soon becomes, under the action of noxious power, highly susceptible of diseased excitement; and, as in the inflammatory affection named gout, it attains to an exquisite degree of pain and acute excitability. Under these circumstances gout is constituted, and characterized by the local symptoms of burning heat, gnawing pain, exquisite sensibility to pressure, tumefaction, efflorescence, shining cuticular distention, and immobility of the affected joint. These appearances will vary in degree, according to the motive conditions of the affected parts, but they will always be sufficiently uniform to exhibit the true character of gouty inflammation.

7. The general symptoms arising from gouty inflammation are those of systematic commotion from sympathetic influence. Much diversity is liable to occur in these general effects on the economy,

nomy, according to the prevailing motive conditions of the system, whether temperamental, habitual, or morbid. When equal energy pervades the frame, with entire freedom from visceral ailment, the diseased agitation will be equally distributed, and not disproportionately arrested on any particular organ, which will afford a general exemption from danger: on the contrary, if stomachic, hepatic, pneumonic, or any other organic affection should exist, the sympathetic effect of the gouty irritation may become preponderant on either of those parts, and induce a higher and more painful degree of visceral disease than would arise from its equal operation; but the gouty patient may even here be consoled, by knowing that the original, as well as the symptomatic affection, is as controllable as common inflammation, between which indeed no essential difference subsists. The cause must be promptly removed; and if the effect should not cease, it must be similarly remedied.

Visceral participation in gouty excitement loses its ideal terror, by rejecting the groundless prejudice by which its quality and danger have been estimated; and, what is of more importance, avoids the greater danger, from the stimulant treatment held to be necessary for the expulsion of gout

from

from the system, whatever may be its supposed situation.

Visceral ailment is always of weighty consideration in the scale of health and life; but it is no small extenuation of the risk to know, that whatever induces inflammation on a vital part, the affection will shape its nature and character to the organ itself, derive no malignancy from the supposed quality of the exciting cause, and become curable by ordinary means of assistance. This is the case of local gout, and every form of its general influence on the system.

If it were an object to combat a name, it may be said that such a term as gout, applied to a visceral part, would be a misnomer, as the structure necessary to its constitution does not exist in the fabric of parts more immediately invested with the function of life.

8. When the onset, as well as developed form of gouty inflammation is connected with much distempered excitability, it will rage with proportionate violence. After establishing itself more particularly on the ligamentous and tendinous structure, it will become first diffused to the surrounding parts, such as the cartilages, perios-

periosteum, bone, and muscle, where the degree of irritation will excite a copious afflux of fluids, and greatly increase the previous pain, by the stimulus of distention.

Parts once in a state of disease are left much to the chance of motive power, whether the con-ditions of health shall be restored, or the organic structure shall so far yield, as to render such an event physically impossible. Animalized matter derives from organic arrangement, active powers, evolvable from, and only tenable with, that peculiar fabric.

A tendency even to deviation from primordial texture is disease, positive change, an incurable grievance. A violent attack, therefore, of gout risks greatly the ultimate integrity of the diseased parts, and endangers leaving an irremediable source of morbid excitability.

The general influence or systematic impression made by gout, will be proportionate to the local affection : when the latter is violent, it forcibly propagates its influence to the system, and there-by reduces' in some measure its concentrated activity on the primarily affected parts.

The

The morbid association of motive power involves every visceral function in risk, in gouty, as in every other description of inflammatory excitement.

There is no foreseeing what organ may more particularly arrest and amass its force; but the hazard of its seriously occurring will depend 'on the violence of the local disease, and the habitual motive conditions of the various organs: if distempered, a promptitude and tenaciousness of morbid impression will exist; on the contrary, if in the firm harmony of health, less susceptibility for diseased change, and less disposition for its continuance, will obtain.

Whatever may be the general effects of gouty irritation, whether they go the length of exciting only a transient agitation throughout the frame, or of generating in any particular organ actual inflammation, it is important to keep incessantly in view, that the curative intention is not varied by the name of the disease, but requires, by its similarity, to be that which is applicable in other inflammatory cases.

9. Diseases arise from the greater or less deviation of motive powers from the standard conditions

tions of health, and are curable or not, according to the degree and nature of the injury sustained. In most instances the inflicted mischief does not incapacitate the aggrieved parts from restoring, by natural effort, the salutary state; and in no disease would spontaneous cure happen more favourably than in gout, if left to its course, unmolested and unperverted by the pernicious treatment of art.

The momentous advantage of obviating the protracted or natural duration of gout, by suitable management, is obvious from the ravage which is made both locally and generally by fostering and aggravating the malady in the accustomed manner.

In opposition to the dictates of common sense, a lengthened fit of the gout is not considered by *reasoning* prejudice as an extension of morbid evil, but, on the contrary, as a remedial good. The Augean stable of medical errors will not b speedily cleansed; but this difficulty should not afford them an unassailable sanctuary.

The parts which are the seat of gouty inflammation are peculiarly liable to irreparable and

truly

truly distressful mischief, from long-continued affection. The ligamentous and tendinous structure will by repeated and delayed irritation soon become impaired in its uniform density, polished surface, cellular flexion, and native excitability; its circulating and exhaling fluids will also suffer in transmission and quality. The confusion resulting from this derangement will generate diseased motions; which, by contiguous sympathy, will proceed to the neighbouring cartilages, periosteum, and bone, inducing distempered action, with its morbid consequences, on the circulating and secreting fluids of those parts.

In this disordered excitability, as well as altered structure, it is not difficult to perceive the cause of the worst effects that characterise prolonged and inveterate gout. If the gouty inflammation be not early subdued, an effusion of coagulable lymph, and a generation of new vessels, will soon permanently thicken and enlarge the affected ligaments and tendons. The continued irritation from this structural derangement will vitiate the vascular action of the periosteal covering of the gouty joint, and force its exhalant vessels to bring back from the bony fabric more or less of ossific principles, with its diluent fluid. These principles are phosphoric

acid

acid and lime, which are combined with other substances, into the form of organic bone, by the nutritive or generative vessels of that structure.

The osseous but unossified substances exhaled on the gouty joint, aggregate, and form in the temperature of the part the calcareous concretions, which, advancing to the cuticular surface by arterial impulse behind, and ulcerative decomposition before, at length appear through the skin, in knots, or tophous tumours, and are finally discharged under the name of chalk-stones.

The stimulant effect of such misplaced substances, the mechanical violence of such rough concretions, and the altered structure of the ligaments and tendons, fill up the measure of deformity and immobility, to which the gouty joint, spoilt by fostered inflammation, is ultimately consigned.

Is all this havock the inevitable progress of the disease, and the irresistible work of Nature?—No: her decrees are not so penal; it is the misdeed of art, resulting from delusive prejudice.

If the more transient form of gouty inflammation should awaken throughout the system
sympathetic irritation, and occasionally overwhelm a vital organ with its preponderant severity, what may not be expected from systematic
and visceral participation, when its long endurance has overspread the constituent parts of the
joint with induration, enlargement, osseous and
other effusions, ulceration, and distention?

These irritating circumstances must violently
influence the motive power of the system, inducing much incessant agitation, extreme indirect debility, and the constant hazard of visceral
inflammation.

The pernicious effect on the systematic health
arising from protracted gout, not only extends
to the general or partial sympathy, which may
be directly induced, but also to the generation of
an habitual facility for morbid impression, which
necessarily leads to frequent disease, and subjects
life itself to a very precarious tenure.

10. The severe effects arising from protracted
gout, clearly evince the urgent necessity for
obviating such mischief by the most prompt and
effectual means of shortening its duration.

The

The chimerical view of constitutional benefit accruing from prolonged or unchecked gout, has fettered every humane attempt to afford seasonable relief, with the clamorous opposition of unfounded prejudice.

The errors of reason debase humanity below the brute creation, by excluding the light of instinct, which is the direct efficiency of physical or innate power, and an unerring guide to rectitude. The disposition which instinct inspires is irresistibly operative, and infallibly commensurate with its object; but wayward and visionary reason, acknowledging no control from facts, no direction from the laws of nature, is the sport of fiction, and the parent of fallacy.

If the gout be early checked, if its worst effects be obviated by a seasonable repression of its force, and curtailment of its duration, the contracted tendon, thickened and indurated ligament, osseous secretion, painful ulceration, rugged enlargement, and irreparable immobility and deformity of the affected joint, may be effectually prevented; and with the avoidance of those local injuries will be connected a constitutional escape from the morbid sympathies, and the

visceral

visceral affections, which lingering and aggravated inflammation is apt to induce.

The cessation of a paroxysm of the gout will be more or less complete in proportion as it has occasioned more or less injury to the affected parts, and associative disturbance to the motive powers of the system. When long delayed, it tends to leave an indelible susceptibility on the affected parts for a renewal of morbid irritation, and to entail a distempered aptitude in the system for participating in the pressure of any occurring malady.

It appears, then, by every well-founded motive of health, by every wish to ward off the inveterate establishment of both local and general disease, that the early removal of gout should be attempted; nor agreeably to a correct view of inflammatory violence, is its existence ever to be endured a moment longer than the inefficacy of the means employed may require; no, not even in conformity to the idle reveries of its being a salutary derivant. No quarter should be given its continuance; it is a growing evil, its delay is dangerous, and its long endurance an irrecoverable mischief.

11. To question the propriety of curing a disease, is surely a solecism in the healing art; but the prevailing opinion of the nature of gout has inveterately opposed the admissibility of attempting to subdue it. Nor will this *morbid prejudice*, in favour of *morbid virtue*, yield the imperial sway which it holds over the medical, as well as popular world, without combating its untenableness, on a ground that will not awaken the alarms of humoral pathology. It is not enough to say that gout is an inflammatory affection, but it is necessary to disembarrass it of every notion of peculiarity of nature, to reconcile the prevailing scientific and public opinion at once to the practicability and expediency of its early cure.

It may then be affirmed, as has been already incidentally observed, that no difference whatever exists between gouty and other forms of inflammation, but in circumstances of degree and situation.

If violence, either from external or internal causes, should derange and excite the motive powers of the ligamentous and tendinous structure, to that painfully active state termed inflammation, appearances will arise correspondent to

the

the common character of that affection; which whether distinguished by the various appellations of gout, rheumatism, sprain, or simple inflammation, the disease is fundamentally the same, the distinction is merely nominal, nor will it be admitted by the most fearfully credulous, that a mere name has magic to conjure up a real difference.

Inflammations of the most specific nature, with respect to cause, such as variolous, vaccine, venereal, scrofulous, cancerous, &c. are perfectly similar in the effect of excessive excitement, and are curable in the same way. The excess is the point of resemblance in external character, and the equal object of cure.

The specific causes of inflammation just recited may be rendered inefficient to that degree of excitement: in that case a morbid, but not an inflammatory action will remain: this is evinced in the systematic diffusion of the variolous, venereal, and other diseases, from local sources.

If the identity of inflammation, under the supposed agency of humoral causes, be admissible, it must be allowed to be at least equally so between the gouty and common description of that

excitement,

citement, in which distempered excitability and external violence are the usual stimulant powers, wholly unaided by the influence of morbid matter.

Inflammatory excitement is universally similar, whatever be its degree or situation. The variety of remote causes, by which it is induced, generates no correspondent difference in its quality. It consists exclusively of active violence. It is a sort of combustive state of vital motion, and may be aptly likened to fire, which, with whatever fuel kindled, burns with identical heat.

12. Gouty inflammation has been variously denominated, according to the tone and situation of the affected part : hence the several terms tonic, atonic, retrocedent, and erratic, or mis-placed gout.

These distinctions are more fanciful than real. They arise from different states of sympathetic energy, and visceral susceptibility for associative or sympathetic impression.

In the unbroken tone, firmness and regularity of motive power is presented an indispensable condition for that violent degree of ligamentous

mentous and tendinous inflammation, which may be truly denominated acute, in reference to its active and rapid nature; in contradistinction to that atonic, enfeebled, and torpid state of motive power, which must necessarily impart to the affection less inflammatory violence, and which may be appropriately named chronic gout, in reference to its comparatively inactive and lingering nature.

In these opposite states of motive power may be recognised two strongly marked characters of gouty malady, descriptively expressed by the terms acute and chronic *. These appellations

at

* The terms acute and chronic, here adopted, signify only different degrees of the same inflammatory affection. They imply no sort of distinction in the quality of the disease, but merely in its quantity, or force. Nor do they involve the gratuitous notion of active and passive inflammation. Animal life itself is constituted by incessant action; its excessive or inflammatory violence, therefore, must necessarily be active. When a vital part is salutarily impressed by agents, it reacts, which produces healthy action; when morbidly impressed, it also reacts, which produces diseased action; but when wholly unimpressed, no action arises, which is death, or the passive state of matter; hence, what is imagined by passive or inactive inflammation, cannot exist compatibly with the organic motion of vital power. If, however, the gouty patient should be at all embarrassed in determining whether an occurring attack should

be

at once respectively denote the force, duration, and radical condition of the disease.

The idea of retrocedent gout is not perfectly correct. When the disease ceases on one joint, the disposition to it on another, either from original or sympathetic susceptibility to be affected, may indeed proceed the length of inflammatory excitement; but this arises entirely from the associated connexion of motive power actuating similar structure, and has less of retrocession or transference, than originality in its nature.

The restricted violence, which gives effect to local disease, by obviating indefinite diffusion, is induced by the derivant, or amassing influence which an aggrieved part exerts on the system generally, and more particularly on kindred structure.

The shifting, or successive attacks of gouty inflammation, impair its concentrated violence,

be referred to the acute or chronic nature, it may be expedient to consult the judgment of a correct and experienced observer of the disease, that all doubt may be removed, as to the degree of inflammation, its concomitant temperature, and how far its reduction should be carried, to ensure the earliest and most effectual cure.

by

by distributing its force. When the affection is extremely vehement, it is often dissipated by extension Its shewing itself, therefore, on different joints, indicates rather a diminution than an augmentation of its force.

Its increasing severity, by undue protraction, subjects it to the slow course of removal which attends its propagation to other joints. Its prompt extinction would be a complete cure, and secure defence from entailing on other joints an active state of the disease.

The retrocession, here considered, implies a distribution of the original disease, and that, instead of being unfavourable, it seems to be the only mode of dispersion which the neglect of early remedy has left.

The erratic, or misplaced gout, has no admissible significancy in either the theory or practice of the disease. It implies visceral or systematic affection, arising from its declining or shifting station on the joints. This resolves itself wholly into the greater or less transient effects of sympathetic irritation,

If,

If, in these circumstances, either the brain or any other vital organ be affected to the extent of inflammatory excitement, the effect will not differ from that of common inflammation. It cannot be what is termed gout, as the brain, as well as every other vital organ, is destitute of the ligamentous and tendinous structure, necessary to that sort of inflammatory affection.

The joints may indeed, in turn, share in the annihilating distribution of inflammatory gout; but it is not probable that such dispersion can excite any morbid irritation on the system, or any of its organs. Whenever these suffer, it is from the vehement pain attending mismanaged and protracted gout.

A long continuance of local pain, whether proceeding from gout or any other cause, tends to exhaust motive energy, to vitiate the conditions of salutary excitability, and to overwhelm the system with an unnatural degree of susceptibility for morbid impression.

Misplaced gout then is a misnomer; when it holds not its natural situation, when it occupies not its indispensable structure, its existence is no where but in branular fiction.

SECTION

SECTION III.

REMOTE AND PROXIMATE CAUSE OF GOUT.

1. Like other diseases, the inflammatory affection termed gout, may be induced by a variety
of causes, operating more or less remotely in
producing the morbid effect.

In the view which has been taken of the nature
and constitution of gout, it occurred to be observed, that the ligamentous and tendinous
structure was the peculiar seat of gouty inflammation. It has been also held that an inflammatory excitement of this fabric is steadily characterized by similar symptoms, however different
the exciting force; whether it be of a physical,
chemical, or mechanical nature, the effect on
the motive power will be the same.

Whatever is capable of inducing painful extension of the ligaments and tendons, is equal
to exciting what is understood by gouty inflammation. External violence in general, but more
particularly that which arises from a sudden and
thwarted

thwarted exertion of the ligaments, tendons, and muscular bandage, or fascia, by stretching them beyond their accustomed and natural dimensions, will occasion much derangement in the healthy fabric of those parts, and consequently a morbid agitation of both the irritative and sentient powers of motion. In these diseased conditions of structure and motive power, may be recognised the true symptoms of gouty inflammation. Exquisite pain, shining tumefaction, articular immobility, and systematic irritation, correctly exhibit the gouty malady: but the sanctioned doctrines of medical schools, as well as popular prejudice, would consider an attempt to assimilate the effects of a sprained joint with gout, as but little short of sacrilegious innovation; as trifling with the holy mistery of inscrutable disease, and rendering great things little indeed. Such declamation may be sounding, but it is nonsensical, without either point or authority, without any just regard for true science and its liberal investigation,

Of what importance to the interest of fair reasoning can it be, to be told, that the subject of inquiry is of vast moment, and should be considered rather with fearful caution than confident freedom? It is not in this way that either

error

error can be detected or truth explained. An examination is surely serious in proportion to the magnitude of its object ; yet, to prove successful, it must be conducted with unyielding firmness, and not with shrinking diffidence.

A mere name is unworthy of dispute, when its object is incontestable. In conformity to this opinion, the epithet gouty is attached to articular inflammation, whether from external or other causes, and denotes the *ideally* dreadful description of disease, that is here reduced to the level of common inflammatory excitement.

When either the ligamentous, tendinous, or fascial structure, is unduly stretched, or sprained, by external violence, such as occurs in wry motion, in jumping and immoderate walking, not only is inflammatory affection the consequence, but the difficulty of effecting a perfect restoration of motive power and energy, in this dense fabric, subjects it to an easy renewal of the injury : hence it is remarkable, that sprained joints are readily excitable, and do, on slight instances of violence, go into actual inflammation, with not only the semblance but acknowledged reality of gout. A sprain is a familiar term, but in its nature it will be found permanently

nently to afford the irritable conditions of frequently recurring inflammation.

If a ligamentous, tendinous, or fascial part be unduly stretched, much lesion of the minute arrangement of that fabric must necessarily happen, to admit of such elongation : this violence may also go the greater degree of lacerating the larger fibres. The vacuities which this derangement makes, are liable to be filled with the generation of new vessels, or organized coagulable lymph. Such mechanical obstacles will occasion morbid thickening, immobility, and excitability in the affected part, which will invite, and facilitate, the future accession of inflammatory or gouty disease.

In the investigation of gouty malady, it is of importance to establish the fact of its being intrinsically and characteristically constituted by inflammatory excitement of ligamentous and tendinous parts, stretching them beyond the bounds of natural motion. This proves that the disease is simple inflammation, resulting from a mechanical cause, and that although either morbid excitability from constitutional causes, or material acrids, may generate a similar excitement,

5   yet

yet that they are not indispensably necessary to the production of the disease.

Rejecting the prevailing opinion, of its being a disease of a specific nature, producible only by its peculiar cause, its contemplation is placed on the broad basis of simple inflammatory affection; acknowledging for its cause every stimulant agency capable of inducing that degree of excitement.

2. External violence inflicted on the ligaments and tendons, by sprain, contusion, or division, is equal to inducing gouty or inflammatory excitement on these parts. The disease in this case results from the direct action of a hurtful power; but another very fertile source of gout is in the spontaneous change that is apt to occur in the vascular fabric of those parts. They are constructed with such minuteness of vessel as to be exanguious, or bloodless, and compacted with such density of cellular and muscular substance, as to lose all appearance of muscularity, and to assume the polished aspect, and firm texture, peculiar to the ligamentous and tendinous structure. Though vessels of sufficient magnitude do not pervade those substances, to admit of the passage of red blood, yet they are

made

made up of transmitting, secreting, exhaling, and nutritive tubes, for the due circulation and uses of the colourless fluids - distributed to them. An interruption of the healthful function of those minute vessels is extremely likely to occur independently of external violence, either from partaking in a morbid state of systematic excitability, or from a local failure of native energy, by which the structure is liable to undergo changes; some of the vessels becoming incapable of transmitting their contents, obstruction, adhesion, and ultimate obliteration of cavity will ensue. This change will cast an additional circulating burden on the adjacent vessels, which, by unduly distending them, will prove a source of inflammatory irritation, assuming more or less the characteristic appearances of gouty excitement, in proportion to the degree of organic derangement, and consequent violence of the affection.

From this cause the disease may be induced in every intermediate degree of force, from a slight gnawing sensation at the depth of the joint, with trifling swelling and efflorescence, to the most racking torture, prominent tumefaction, and calcareous deposition.

The

The origin of gout from morbid changes in the vascular structure, and function of the ligaments and tendons, occurs more particularly in the decline of life, from fifty to sixty years of age. At that time vital energy begins to droop, and exposes the various excitability of different parts to morbid affection, and more especially the ligamentous and tendinous fabric, which, from being almost incessantly occupied in locomotive exertion, is peculiarly liable to the complicated injuries of attrition, indirect debility, and morbid excitement.

Under these circumstances, the disease arises without hereditary predisposition; and, like the origin from external violence, it owes its existence to accidental influence.

3. However gouty inflammation may have been repeatedly produced, whether by external violence, the gradual formation of altered structure, or local excess of distempered excitability on the ligamentous, tendinous, and fascial parts, the morbid changes induced, will at length become so radically influential in the motive powers of the system, as to generate a transmittable state of temperamental susceptibility for morbid affection. The offspring in such diseased circum-

stances,

stances, will possess constitutional powers equal to the ordinary functions of health, but yet accompanied with a temperamental disposition to the disease. In these instances gouty excitability may be said to be hereditary. The motive powers of the system at large have an undue excess of impressibility, while those of the ligamentous and tendinous structure are subjected to it in a preponderant degree. These intrinsically morbid conditions may never go the length of actual disease, if causes sufficiently excitant do not operate on the native susceptibility for being affected. Thus it often occurs that the progeny of gouty parents is exempt from the formal attack of the disease, neither external injuries, nor the internal conditions of health, having furnished exciting causes sufficient to induce ligamentous or tendinous inflammation.

Hereditary liability to this affection is very much under the control of an abstemious mode of living, with respect to diet and fermented liquors, regular temperature and moderate exercise. If due regard be paid to these important conditions of health, neither an inherent disposition to gout, nor its originating causes, will be often sufficiently operative to develope that malady.

As

As generation is not the work of disease, but that of health; the powers of incipient life oppose an early and progressive resistance to the growth of morbid organization. Nor indeed would the phenomena of vitality be compatible with the degree of disease that could be formally active at the commencement of organic arrangement: hence it rarely occurs, that the fœtal state partakes of maternal contagion, even in variolous, venereal, or other contaminating maladies.

The providence of nature is strikingly manifested in the repugnance which is shewn to the hereditary transmission of diseases, by limiting the capability of imparting them in this way to a condition of organic power, that seems to be radically founded in deficient energy or tone, and that never can discover more than a disposition or morbid susceptibility for proceeding to actual disease, on the application of adequate exciting causes.

This doctrine is not confined to gouty inflammation, but is universally applicable to all hereditary affections. Thus the scrofulous disease is founded in a morbidly weak and irritable temperament, preponderating on the lymphatic and

glandular

glandular structure; the maniacal, on that of the nerves predominant on the brain.

These diseases never arise naturally, and probably never would be evolved or realized, if the vitiating influence of intemperate diet and irregular exertion did not force them into actual existence.

The gouty habit or susceptibility is the same, whether native or induced, and is evinced by a promptitude to ligamentous and tendinous inflammation. The conditions upon which this liability rests, being founded in morbid excitability, may subject the general health to various forms of molestation, according to the respective state and habitude of the different organs. A febrile commotion may fundamentally and universally shake the fabric of health; inflammatory action, equally pervading the system, may do the same; while a more insulated disturbance on either of the organs would have an appropriate, but less general influence.

The diseases which may arise to the general health, under natural circumstances of distempered excitability of the system, predominantly existing on any of the vital organs, have no identity,

tity, nor even relevancy to gouty excitement, which requires as an indispensable condition to its existence, the presence of either the ligamentous or tendinous fabric. It is erroneous therefore to say, that gout is afloat in the system, when either the general or visceral health is distempered. The idea is a fiction, aiming to embody a nonentity. Let the accidental affection of general health be significantly denominated, according to its particular nature, but suffer not the inflammatory excitement of a peculiar structure to be synonimous with every form and degree of morbid irritation, which may arise in the general system. Nor must gouty excitement, or ligamentous and tendinous inflammation, be considered as curative of systematic diseases.

That a greater evil diverts the attention from a less, is a fact of incessant experience, both in the physical and moral world; but that an addition of a most painful and violent disease should be considered as salutary, would be reasoning, as well as acting, through a very diseased medium, and would involve a paradox, at once repugnant to common sense and the axioms of efficient quantity.

E 3

The

The attempt at curing one disease by the substitution of another, has in general more of an aggravating, than of an alleviating tendency. The newly instituted disease must be the more powerful to be curative; and would not this be literally realizing the medicinal injury of rendering the remedy worse than the disease?

Topical irritation often indeed operates salutarily derivant from the system, when visceral excitement oppresses and endangers a vital function. This benefit may be suitably rendered by vesication, pustulation, and rubefacience; but it will hardly be judged either safe, or consistent with this revulsive principle, to bruise, sprain, or wound a ligament or tendon, with a view to beneficial excitement. Until this be thought vindicable practice, the occurrence of gouty inflammation, which would be similar violence, must be rather deprecated than desired.

4. A morbid susceptibility on the ligamentous and tendinous parts, for diseased action, has been seen to be derivable from external violence, spontaneous defection of vascular structure, and hereditary transmission. Other causes may occur to produce this painful distemper. Among these

these prominently presents variable temperature, inducing catarrhal affection, and an unequal distribution of the circulating fluids. The diseased irritation, which results from the stimulus of morbid distention, when the balance of the circulating fluids is deranged, may be felt in various parts of the system, and speedily on the ligaments and tendons, if they should have previously suffered from inflammatory violence; and even if the promptitude for diseased impression connected with former ailment should not exist, yet it will always be possible, though much less probable, that changes in temperature, inducing catarrhal disease, may be determined to the usual seat of gouty inflammation.

Frequent colds, independently of the co-operative influence of local changes, tend to induce the irritation termed rheumatic, which has been said to be a modification only of gouty excitement. The frequent renewal of that affection will afford equal certainty and celerity to its production, on the occurrence of catarrhal commotion.

Hence is seen another way, in which gouty inflammation may be induced, not only by the influence of temperature, when morbid suscep-

tibility

tibility for diseased action has been generated in the ligamentous and tendinous structure, from former suffering, but also of its competency, gradually to effect those changes, either by the undue stimulating agency of excessive distention, or the direct transference of diseased irritation.

The issue of that systematic affection which an irregular distribution of the circulating fluids induces from unsteady temperature, must be necessarily precarious. It is usually indeed determined to the tracheal and bronchial structure, both from an impediment to equal circulation speedily surcharging the lungs, and from natural consent subsisting between pulmonary and cuticular exhalation.

The healthy balance of those outlets depends on each course sharing them in a just proportion. If deficient excretion occurs at the skin, a morbid push will be made on the bronchial and tracheal membrane, to reject by that route the redundant determination, while excessive perspiration induces diseased dryness of the bronchial, tracheal, and fauceal membrane, with consequent thirst, cough, and difficult respiration. But the effects of irregular circulation are not always shewn in this

this form : any other organ may, and often is, either originally or sympathetically affected.

There is not a function in the animal economy, from that of the brain, to the secretion of mucus for lubricating surfaces, but what may be disturbed by the influence of reduced heat, in diminishing cuticular excretion. The effect may be aptly compared to what would arise from the suppression of the steam of hot water : in that case, heat is retained, instead of escaping in aqueous vapour ; so in the animal system, the heat which should be incessantly dissipating by the evaporation of redundant fluid, will be partly retained, and molest both by excess in quantity and temperature.

Every instance then of suppressed perspiration furnishes in a greater or less degree the stimulant powers of excessive heat and vascular distention. In whatever parts these noxious agents may happen to be disproportionately amassed, much violent excitement must ensue. The ligaments and tendons are not exempt from this determination of morbid agency, and do often afford striking examples of its influence in violent inflammatory affection. The practical worth of these reflections on the effects of

variable

variable temperature, consists in clearly cata-
loguing gouty inflammation with the common
effects of disturbed circulation, and thereby
to assimilate both its nature and cure; to that
which is applicable to catarrhal, or to other
local or general inflammatory affection.

5. It has been observed, that the undue distention occurring in particular parts of the frame,
from an unequal distribution of the circulating
fluids, is a fertile cause of morbid excitement :
on the same principle, a surcharge of fluidity
in the system, from full diet and inaction, tends
to produce similar effects.

The exigencies of health require a certain
proportion of nutriment, which indeed will vary
according to temperamental and habitual circumstances. A given quantity of food may
be said to be sufficient, if an early habit should
have been established of taking no more: from
that, would result the vascular tension, and
motive energy, necessary to a full exertion of
animal power; but if a larger portion should
have been usually taken, so as to plead the influence of custom for its continuance, it may be
unsafe to resist this claim, by what may be
thought an adequate standard allowance.

4

But

But though some diversity and difficulty necessarily present in adjusting the salubrious measure of nutriment, in different temperamental and habitual circumstances, none can exist, as to the universal necessity of regulating its amount by the degree of bodily exertion which may be made. Here nature seeks an indemnity against all irregularities; and when they are not extravagantly indulged, an efficacious remedy is found in a suitable degree of exercise.

The voluntary motions of the body increase all the secretions and excretions; they dissipate also the motive power of vital action, and thereby at once obviate morbid plenitude, and induce that salutary inanition which imperiously demands supply by hunger, or appetite for taking food.

This natural call to recruit exhausted power, farther ensures a due assimilation of what is taken, both by the perfect quality of the gastric fluid, or digestive solvent, secreted in the stomach, and the vigorous action which will be exerted by that organ, and the intestines, on what is swallowed, for its alimentary conversion.

The

The lacteal vessels will then secrete from this chylous matter its most nutritive parts, and animalize them in such a way, as to fit them to be incorporated and consolidated in the various structure of the animal frame. This alimentary process will proceed for some time without the healthful influence of exercise; but as it tends to oppress by plenitude, it must be considered as paving the way to the various affections which may originate from such morbid distention.

In this variety of malady, the stomach is likely to be in the van of suffering; its frequent incumbrances impair its motive energy, vitiate its solvent secretion, and awaken throughout the system sympathetic participation in its grievance.

The stomach may be considered as the common centre of excitability, from whence issues, in numberless ramifications, its associated connexion with the whole system: this organ therefore suffers either originally or sympathetically in every disease that materially disturbs the functions of health.

The important share which the stomach has, both as an excitable and alimentary organ, in the

the maintenance of life and health, evinces the necessity of not oppressing it, either by the direct effect of indulging in immoderate meals, or in indolently neglecting such exercise as would prevent systematic plenitude.

In circumstances of personal inability for exercise, the quantity of nutriment should be proportionately diminished, and the portion taken at a time, should be so small as never to endanger stomachic oppression.

With the plenitude resulting from dietetic excess and deficient exercise, are allied the various morbid effects of immoderate distentions in different parts of the system; on the brain, inducing headach; the lungs, cough; stomach, imperfect digestion; bowels, inflammation and flatulence; and kidneys, diseased irritation, with irregular secretion of urine; on the womb, hysteric affection, with disordered menstruation; and on the ligamentous and tendinous structure, gouty or inflammatory excitement,

The frequency of gouty disease, in connexion either with systematic plenitude, or morbid excitability of the stomach, consequent on dietetic excess, strongly marks the liability the
ligaments

ligaments and tendons are under, of participating in the diseased irritation, induced either by undue distention or sympathetic influence.

The familiar occurrence of these associated affections has also induced the prevailing opinion, that dyspeptic, and other disorders of the stomach, are often of gouty origin, and are salutarily expelled to the joints, from whence, if not duly stationed, they may return, and take the stomach by surprise. This is the gouty patient's jeopardy, and indeed, to the utter disgrace of medical science, the grave amount of ancient and modern speculation on the subject, to the instant of the present inquiry. The theory of the disease here submitted to the public, renounces all credit in such imaginary and groundless danger. The stomach may indeed sympathize with inflamed ligaments and tendons, in every degree of violence, from transient pain to positive inflammation ; but then the sympathy will not have transferred either ligament or tendon to the stomach, and of course cannot have endued it with the physical possibility even of being affected with gouty inflammation : whatever therefore may be its sympathetic affection, it must be treated in a

manner

manner appropriate to its own power and structure, without any reference to the chimerical notions of the remedial nature of gout.

Gouty excitement is peculiar to the ligamentous and tendinous structure; it therefore can have no place in the stomach, brain, bowels, or any of the visceral parts; and if it can only affect those organs, by the sympathetic influence of local pain, such as would be occasioned by a wound, fracture, and other external violence, the disease will be stripped of its ideal terrors, assume its painful, but in no other respect dangerous station, on the ligamentous and tendinous structure, as being exclusively, peculiarly, and indispensably necessary to its existence.

6. The morbid irritation which may arise either generally, or locally, from plenitude and inaction, may be also induced by the undue stimulant influence of immoderate indulgence in fermented liquors. It is impossible, but the motive conditions of health must be distempered by the violent agitation induced by the abuse of excitant fluids. The hurtful impression they occasion, is first felt in the general exhaustion of healthful strength, primarily denoted by

by unsteadiness in every motion; then, tremor; and, if life should long enough endure, ultimately by palsy.

This change from the healthy state may be defined debility, not resulting from the abstraction of excitement, as in direct weakness, but from its excessive application, so that it is of an indirect nature, or produced through the medium of immoderately exerted power.

This enfeebled state presents a deplorable susceptibility for diseased impression of every kind. The morbidly agitated and sentient fibre throughout the system, promptly assumes every variety of disease which exciting causes may be adapted to produce. Indigestion, headach, palpitation, and nephritic pain, usually precede either the determination or developement of distempered excitement on the ligaments and tendons. When an impression is produced in the gouty form, other diseased feelings and symptoms vanish, in comparative consideration, though in reality no benefit is commonly afforded; indeed, in proportion to the violence and duration of the gouty pain, will be the degree of general disorder of the system. Accelerated pulse, loss of appetite, disturbed

disturbed secretions and excretions, with excessive temperature, will mark the constitutional connexion which is held with the local pain.

Gouty inflammation occurring in the indirect debility induced by intemperate drinking, is of an inveterate and dangerous nature, from the radical difficulty of restoring the motive conditions of health, and the sympathetic violence which may arise in any of the vital organs. Its danger therefore should be correctly estimated, and the avoidance of its cause proportionately regarded.

The fact of hard drinkers being scourged by this malady, even to the severity of martyrdom itself, has been attested through all ages, from remote antiquity; which at once evinces the pernicious effects of such practice, and the nature of the mischief it induces in the motive powers of health.

It is difficult to imagine a more harassing and precarious tenure of life, than that which presents in the demolished strength, vitiated excitability, and prompt aptitude for diseased impression, occurring in the tremulous bacchanalian. He exhibits a fearful picture of agitated

F   life,

life, prepared to catch the impression of any disease which accidental causes may excite. In such dying circumstances, can it be wondered, that the full form of gouty excitement can scarcely obtain?

The ligaments and tendons may indeed be stimulated, their motive power may be agitated, and the uneasiness of morbid distention may be produced; but every changing condition in such debility is too fugitive, and too incapable of fixation, to give characteristic effect to any description of malady.

Gouty affections in hard drinkers are accordingly remarkable for being transient and undecided, and often embarrass both the medical practitioner and patient with unfounded anxiety for the consequences of the disease not making a more regular and durable appearance.

As rationally may it be expected that either a mortified or paralytic part would spontaneously evolve inflammatory action, as that gout should formally and permanently obtain in such inadequate circumstances for its production.

7. It

7. It must be obvious from what has been observed, that the systematic excitability may be disordered in various ways, and that, from either general or associative connexion, the motive power of the ligamentous and tendinous structure may be excited to acute inflammation.

In the list of remote causes of gout, diminished secretions and suppressed excretions are prominently operative. Scanty secretions of urine and perspiration principally disturb the harmony of health, by inducing stimulant redundancy of the circulating fluids; but a deficient secretion of bile, pancreatic juice, or of mucus, as well as suppression of piles, or any other habitual discharge, whether from ulcer or any other source, will also encumber the vascular system with morbid distention, which either by equal participation, or preponderance, may induce gouty inflammation of the ligaments and tendons.

The secreting and excreting offices of life are only duly performed when the nicest balance of healthful energy pervades the system. If either general or particular excitability should be distempered, some secretion, with its correspondent excretion, will become more or less

deranged,

deranged, and prove a source of growing and extensive disorder. It is not then extraordinary that ligamentous and tendinous excitability should be stimulated to inflammatory or gouty affection, by a failure in the urinary, perspirable, bilious, or any other secretion.

8. It has been seen that habitual indigestion acts as a powerful remote cause of gouty affection. Its mischievous influence is much increased by its frequent alliance with imperfect chylification and costiveness.

The want of renewed energy, which an inadequate formation of chyle necessarily occasions, must speedily be felt in every function of life, and in every action of health. Vital motion will soon be radically affected, and its distempered influence be universally evident.

Costiveness, or torpid action of the peristaltic motion of the intestines, is in the train of the systematic injury sustained by insufficient chyle, which serves to interrupt the course of the circulating fluids; and thus to superadd the noxious effects of partial distention, to the languor and inanity of deficient nutriment.

An

An imperfect chylification may injure the alimentary canal, by inducing morbid excitement; but it debilitates the system, by withholding from lacteal secretion the necessary supply for the ulterior purpose of nutriment. An imperfect chyle indeed cannot find admission through the lacteal vessels. An arranging effect is produced in the transmission through them, which renders to the system the genuine principles of nutriment : thus, it is the deficient quantity, and not the vitiated quality of aliment, that impairs the general health, under circumstances of unduly prepared chyle.

A want of stomachic energy and adequate solvent power in the gastric fluid, are the ground of imperfect chylification in every instance; but default in systematic nutriment is often referable either to glandular obstruction of the mesentery, or to such a distempered state of the motive power of the lacteal vessels, as incapacitates them for a healthful or nutritive secretion.

These causes, so destructive to systematic strength, so productive of diseased excitability, occasionally exert in a very signal manner their

influence

influence in inducing inflammatory or gouty affection of the ligaments and tendons.

The aged, and scrofulous, seem to be more particularly liable to have gouty ailment excited in this way: hence the affection is seldom very distinct; transient pains in the joints are sympathetically distributed over the frame, either without any inflammatory action, or in so feeble a degree, as scarcely to cause perceptible swelling or redness.

In these circumstances, much alarm is usually entertained for the lurking danger which is supposed to be in the rear of imperfect gout; indeed solicitude for the darling remedy, the curative disease, not unfrequently goes the preposterous length of applying topical excitement to the painful joint, in the ardent but delusive hope of there erecting and stationing the sure bulwark of health.

However far-fetched the attempt, medical ingenuity, or rather medical *placebo*, may not be wanting, in endeavouring to relieve indigestion, imperfect chylification, and habitual costiveness, by blistering or otherwise stimulating the feet; but it would exceed even such a view of salutary

tary

tary derivancy, to think of exciting an inflammation on the ligamentous and tendinous structure. The supervening pain would speedily engage a farther effort to allay such intolerable torture, by the aid of poultices and anodynes. That which would then be so egregiously absurd in correct explanation, is held to be vindicable, is indeed supposed to be indispensable, when obscured by the humoral nonsense, and ghostly dread of recondite gout.

The barter of diseases is at best an equally speculative and precarious traffic; and, if ever negotiable, could not be extended to gout on common parity of advantage; for what disorder that could be alleviated by the derivant influence of gouty inflammation, could occasion more local torture, and systematic commotion, than such violence on the ligamentous and tendinous structure?

9. When occasional derangement of health, from whatever cause, has so vitiated the systematic excitability, as universally to awaken a morbid susceptibility for being impressed by noxious powers, gouty, or ligamentous and tendinous inflammation must ever be an impending evil: thus, the frequent recurrence of

febrile

febrile and catarrhal affection, protracted indigestion, habitual intemperance and costiveness,
are among the foremost of the remote causes
which introduce gouty disease.

In these circumstances, the disorder steals into
form very insidiously; disease previously pervades the system, no part or function is entirely
free from unhealthy movement; but often without there being any established character of
malady, gouty inflammation becomes prominent, and at once gives name and definite appearance to the complaint.

The arrival of gout in this manner is wel-
comed with much joy, the disease is held to
be salutary, and undue confidence in its real
and fictitious influence concenters every pain,
every ailment, in this curative disorder. Nor is
the delusion removed by either the continuance
of severe symptoms of the previous systematic
affection, or by the sympathetic disturbance induced by the now local source of irritation.

In such distempered state of excitability, an
aptitude is afforded to every variety of disease,
and especially to gouty excitement, as the ligamentous and tendinous structure must necessarily
share

share a large proportion of the irritative and sentient irregularity which pervades the system, both from its dense fabric and motive uses.

10. Whatever may have first induced gouty inflammation, whether it may have originally participated in the general state of the system, or have been more directly excited by external violence, its having had an existence facilitates its renewal, which disposition at length attains to habitual ease.

Like most diseases connected with impaired tone or energy in the affected parts, the tendency in gout to return increases in the ratio of its actual recurrence. The oftener it has been renewed, the more familiar and frequent will be its visits. In this respect it obeys a law of the animal economy, that subjects every vital, as well as salutary movement, to the influence of custom; and it is by this aid that perfection is ultimately attained, both in the physical and moral world.

An engine so powerful as that of habit, may be wielded to the most salutary as well as morbid purposes, in the various ordinances of life. If not of a salutary tendency, it should be resisted before

fore it shall have acquired, from long continuance, the inveteracy of unyielding establishment. The endeavour at this counteraction is
favoured by the difficulty of subduing the native
energy, which opposes the usurping infringement of habitual power. With such aid, no
quarter should be given, obstacles should be
thickly planted against such ascendancy, which
would hold it in check, and eventually turn the
force of habit to the protection of original
power.

The expediency of this conflict is generally
admissible in diseases, but more particularly so in
gouty inflammation, which tends rapidly to induce such changes in the excitable powers and
organic structure of the affected parts, as greatly
strengthen the disposition to habitual establishment,

No disease, has given more glaring proof of
the facility and obstinacy with which it familiarly
inmates itself, than gout; nor is there any disease
short of visceral lesion, either of more troublesome tenantry, or more frequently rebellious.
It soon takes the lead of systematic ailment; and
when the general health is unoffended, and has
extended no generative sympathy to the peculiar

seat

seat of its violence, it will arise spontaneously, or at least without any other cause than that which habitual promptitude for affection furnishes.

The prevailing pathological notion of the nature of gout, has most perniciously warranted its being fostered. Hailed as a remedial good, it is nursed from pigmy to gigantic power; nor is this cherishing encouragement withheld until it shall have fashioned the affected parts to the prompt acceptance and lasting duration of its violence.

Instead of this procedure, its continuance should be efficaciously resisted, its attack should incite the terror due to an insidious, increasing, and formidable disease, tending at once to erect for itself in the damaged fabric of the ligaments and tendons a familiar and permanent dwelling, and from thence to impair the energy of life, and disconcert the harmony of health, by sympathetically diffusing over the system morbid irritation.

Habitual gout then is habitual disease, often indeed irresistible from altered structure in the
affected

affected parts, but always of hurtful tendency, and therefore should, if possible, be invariably counteracted, and its attacks combated by the most prompt and effectual modes of relief.

11. The proximate cause of gout results from the aggregate efficiency of the remote causes, and is truly the disease itself. This efficiency or proximate cause, by which the disease is constituted, consists in an agitated and an increased degree of vital or repulsive motion in the affected parts.

By vital motion is meant a repellency, subsisting between the constituent particles of all matter. This innate power or property is, by a law of nature, spontaneously evolved from atomical surfaces, and assumes character and determinal force, when issuing from the congeries, or combination of material substances, which forms specific or particular structure.

The exertion of this universally repellent power, in the organic fabric of the animal economy, is life, or vital motion. The action of this power denotes itself in animal feeling as heat; an undistinguishable identity, therefore,

with

with respect to the object, subsists between what has been variously denominated repulsive motion, vital action, and heat. These several modes of the same thing arise from the different circumstances in which it is operative. Repulsive motion is the natural efficiency of matter, and universally pervades every conceivable atom; vital motion is the organic efficiency of matter, and heat is the impression only, which that power makes on animal sensation.

In this view of the nature of vital power, it will be easy to perceive the ground of its morbid excitement in gouty inflammation, as well as in every other variety of disease; it also instructively developes and explains the real cause of all the distressing torture occurring in inflammatory gout, to consist in almost a combustive degree of redundant heat, or repulsive motion. The definition, therefore, here submitted, of the proximate cause of gout being a morbid excess of heat, is perfectly consonant with the explanation offered, of the nature and origin of that power.

The utmost practical advantages are likely to ensue from contemplating the foundation of gout, in common with all other diseases, as laid in
repulsive

repulsive motion, and of assimilating this innate property of matter with the cause of heat *.

In this identity is presented an easy solution of the various intricate questions which have agitated and divided the schools of medicine, from the remotest periods to the present time; and, what is of still greater importance, it leads very directly to an appropriate, and consequently to a successful mode of cure.

Gouty inflammation affords a most striking example, unique indeed in the catalogue of diseases, how much the general theory and practice of medicine promise to be benefited by the explanation here given of its proximate cause. It at once rejects the unmeaning doctrines which issued from the reveries of humoral pathology,

---

* My earliest independent speculations on the nature of disease (now nearly twenty years since) were founded on temperature and its occasional variations. The obvious expansions and contractions which accompany increased and diminished heat, were, in my judgment, of the most extensive and important application in the doctrine and cure of diseases. But the theory of repulsive motion, as explained by the ingenious Mr. Humphrey Davy (in his Essay on Heat, Light, &c.), in rejection of material heat, has contributed greatly to elucidate and confirm my previous view of the subject.

and

and points out an infallible mode of relief, and often indeed of perfect cure.

Gouty excitement, in common with that of every other description, is chiefly cognisable by the greater or less degree of heat which accompanies it : this therefore is an agitated, and consequently an excessive evolution of vital motion, endeavouring to escape by the affected part, torturing the sentient fibre by its accumulated force, and requiring the coldest media for its speedy and curative transference.

As vital motion, in healthy as well as morbid states, is generated by the atomical and compound efficiency of organic matter, its excess, defect, and diseased agitation, must depend on the existing motive conditions of the animal fabric.

Augmented or disturbed action invariably evolves a proportionately increased degree of repulsive motion, correctly noticeable by the impression of excessive heat, which it makes on the sensorial principle of life.

The healthy state of vital motion is liable to be disturbed by an infinity of remote causes, in the

the excitant action of all which, either a painful
or heated sensation is induced, which serves to
mark morbid deviation from the standard temperature; and though excessive heat should not
be thermometrically discoverable at the surface,
yet it actually prevails, as the necessary effect of
commotion; and its dissipation, or transference, by cooling means, will most effectually
restore the motive power to the duly repulsive or
healthy harmony.

When the vital power of the system is deficient, it is designated by correspondent chilliness
and torpor, approaching in some instances even
to paralytic affection; but this can never be an
object for discrimination in gouty ailment: there
the inflammatory heat faithfully characterizes the
excess of vital motion, and correctly points out
the true intention of cure.

SECTION

SECTION IV.

CURE OF GOUT.

1. THE importance of correctly knowing the proximate cause of a disease (which is in fact the disease itself), is evident, in suggesting an appropriate and efficacious mode of cure.

The misconception of the nature of a disorder leads to an erroneous practice, and sanctions the worst consequences by doctrinal prescription.

It would be better for the interests of humanity that no theory of disease should exist, than that the authority derived from it should induce a disregard to facts, and trammel the curative plan with the heedless procedure of routine treatment.

Gouty excitement, whether it proceeds the length of inflammation, or to that only of diseased irritation, affords by its nature, or proximate cause, a striking example of the only suitable mode of cure. This must consist in

G   both

both the local and general diminution of the excessive heat which prevails.

Until this shall have been effected, not a truce even can be gained with the disease ; it must proceed unchecked, and produce locally, as well as generally, all the ravage which its unmitigated violence and protracted duration can occasion. It is obvious that the indication for reduced heat must be regulated, as to its extent, by the subsisting degree of inflammation and pain.

These symptoms must be relieved, and the power of the means for effecting it must be commensurate with the difficulty of the accomplishment.

2. This curative reduction of morbid excess of heat, in gouty disease, is most commodiously and effectually attainable, by the employ of cold media, to transfer the redundant temperature with the utmost dispatch.

Cold water is the universal boon of nature, is the vehicle of atmospheric temperature, in which the functions of health are carried on, and to the refrigerant offices of which, intemperate heat yields its hurtful influence. The fluid then, which

which bears this salutary temperature, is the simple and efficacious remedy here proposed, for the immediate relief and speedy cure of gouty in common with every description of inflammation. It should be applied topically to the affected parts, either by means of wetted cloths, by gentle showering, or actual immersion. A durable degree of cold must be supported; the refrigerant force, therefore, of its first application must be uniformly continued, by frequently renewing the cold water, which soon becomes heated by the inflammatory temperature of the affected parts. This course should be pursued until the painful sensation of burning heat shall subside, and with it the concomitant efflorescence and tumefaction.

It cannot be determined with any precision, that could be even generally applicable, how long this refrigerating treatment should be continued; but an unerring practical rule may be drawn from the attendant heat and pain, which is, unremittedly to persist in the remedy until every sense of painful heat be completely subdued, and the affected parts begin to regain motive power.

If

If a general period can be given, in which curative benefit is derivable from the employ of this simple remedy, it may be fixed at *forty-eight hours*; but for the consolation of the patient be it known, that relief is coeval with its first use, and uninterruptedly progressive to its ultimate completion.

Much will depend on the unveering uniformity with which this remedy is applied. It should not be forgotten that the object to be effected is literally the extinction of fire; and that, therefore, it would not be less unwise to desist before its accomplishment, than it would be to check only, or repress, the conflagration of a building, instead of completely annulling it.

As gouty excitement is kindled only by excessive heat, it is solely this exuberance that is the object of reduction. As soon as that is effected, the topical cold which had fulfilled the intention should be discontinued, lest it might impair the vital energy of the parts, by transferring too much of its motive or salutary heat.

Entire freedom from pain, from inordinate heat, and the renovated sensations of health, will

truly

truly attest an adequate and curative reduction of the morbid temperature.

In the northerly, and indeed in the European latitudes, the topical use of water, at the atmospheric temperature, will be in general found fully sufficient to transfer the redundant heat of gouty inflammation ; though inveterate cases should certainly be combated with either ice or snow, the solution of which on the affected parts would most powerfully operate in reducing the distempered heat *.

In the equinoctial latitudes, or tropical climates, the low temperature of ice or snow would detach from the inflamed parts much more promptly and efficaciously than the temperate coldness of water, at the atmospheric heat,

---

* In default of ice or snow, the atmospheric temperature of water may be reduced upwards of ten degrees of Fahrenheit's thermometer, by dissolving in it one eighth part of the nitrate of potash (common nitre). With this solution the inflamed parts may be wetted instead of common water.

The rapid evaporability of æther at the inflammatory temperature renders it likewise a topical refrigerant of considerable power, and worthy of co-operative employ in those rare, those almost inconceivable cases indeed, which may require the collective force of various means to reduce the morbid heat.

could

could possibly do. The more powerful remedy therefore should be occasionally resorted to *.

The efficacy of topical cold, in gouty inflammation, is much assisted by internal dilution with cold slender liquids, particularly water, drank in small quantities, at short intervals.

* As it is almost impracticable either to transport or to preserve the frozen texture in the shape of snow or ice in the high temperature of the tropical climates, a degree of cold commensurate with every exigence for adequately reducing the morbid heat of gouty inflammation, may be obtained by dissolving muriate of ammonia (ammonia muriata) and nitrate of potash (kali nitratum), each one part, in three parts of water. The solution or distribution of the concrete particles of these saline substances will engage so large a portion of the heat, or repulsive motion of the water, as to reduce its temperature from fifty to ten degrees of Fahrenheit's thermometer, which is twenty-two degrees below the freezing point, by the same scale.

This would be a diminution of heat equal to every salutary purpose of topical cold, much too great indeed, but for cases which may resist a more moderate temperature, and never applicable but with the most exact caution of discontinuing it as soon as the painful sense of morbid heat shall subside, lest the vital action of the affected part should be suspended, or even destroyed by it. Much lower degrees of heat may be induced by the frigorific effect resulting from the commixture of snow, the neutral salts, and mineral acids, in certain proportions; but the influence of such combinations on the animal fibre is not compatible with life.

A common

A common wine-glassful of cold water, taken every ten minutes, soon diffuses a most pleasing refrigerant influence over the system, removes the cuticular constriction, which proceeds from redundant heat, and consequently induces the additionally cooling process of equable perspiration, by which excessive heat is farther evaporated, and the healthy temperature speedily restored. To co-operate in this cooling plan, dietetic and medicinal stimulants should be carefully avoided. Fermented liquors of every kind should be shunned, and but a very moderate quantity of animal food should be taken. The quantity of aliment should never be sufficient to cause either stomachic oppression or dyspeptic excitement: costiveness should be removed, and the apartment should be well ventilated, be without fire, and cautiously kept at the lowest atmospheric temperature. The bed-clothes should be light, and every description of mental anxiety should be solicitously guarded against.

Both the local and general mode of reducing morbid heat, here recommended, must be understood to be as strictly applicable to every shifting or sympathetic attack, on a fresh joint, as to the original seizure.

It

It is also to be remembered, that the success of the treatment will be earlier and more decisive, if topical cold be applied at the same time, and in an equal degree, to every part which may happen to be affected, whether in the first instance, successively, or interchangeably.

This refrigerant mode of cure is of course indicated in every inflammatory gradation of gouty, or ligamentous and tendinous excitement, usually termed rheumatism, but which has been before said to be a misnomer, and to hold the strictest identity with the more evident character of gout.

3. But little assistance can be derived from medical influence in the cure of gouty affection; and indeed but little occasion can occur for its aid, if the full effect of reduced temperature, both locally and generally, has been obtained. The violent local pain, and symptoms of general irritation, usually attending a high degree of gouty excitement, cannot fail to impair the systematic energy extremely, and even dangerously, if long protracted.

The removal of these evils should be attempted without the shortest delay; to endure them is to

tamper

tamper with the interests of health, and to compromise the existence of a most distressing and threatening malady. Reduced temperature, adequately applied, will, in a vast majority of instances, effectually remedy every grievance, and leave nothing for medicinal assistance to accomplish.

In the few cases which may occur of unyielding torture, arising from deeply altered structure in the affected parts, deranged distribution of circulating fluids, and extreme temperamental irritability, aid may be sought for in the harmonizing efficacy of opium, and other narcotics. It has been my practice occasionally to direct the camphorated tincture of opium (tinctura opii camphorata), and the ammoniated tincture of guaiacum (tinctura guaiaci ammoniata), in doses from one dram to half an ounce of each, in any suitable vehicle, at intervals of four hours; but this in most instances has been rather the work of medical expediency, to gratify the prevailing expectation of something medicinal being necessary, than from a clear persuasion of its being indispensably requisite. In the worst cases, where pain has been insufferable, the topical application of cold has afforded immediate relief, and its constant employ during some

hours

hours has obviated the recurrence of farther in-convenience. In similar instances, opium in the largest doses, without refrigerant co-opera-tion, has not availed in rendering the pain even tolerable, much less in wholly removing it.

The proximate cause of gouty excitement consisting in excessive heat, or repulsive motion, amassed and confined in the dense structure of the ligaments and tendons, affords a satisfactory explanation of the inefficacy of opiate or narcotic influence in allaying the pain. The solitary action of that power must tend to increase rather than diminish its violence, by exciting additional motive energy in the affected parts *,

which

* Opium is here considered as a *narcotic stimulant*, in decided opposition to its supposed claim to a direct sedative power. Such ideal power, indeed, implies negation or abstraction of all positive power, which is repugnant to every effect induced by opium on animal excitability. Diminished frequency of arterial action certainly arises from its influence; but how is this produced ? not by suspending or repressing motive power, but by so exciting and invigorating it, as to render its contractile actions propor-tionately more strong, equal, and slow. This retarded fre-quency of action then results from the improved tone and regu-larity imparted by opiate or narcotic excitement, which effectually supersede the agitated, rapid, and irregular motions of debility. Hence the injurious effects induced by the stimulating influence of opium in inflammatory and other diseases of high excitement, and its beneficial agency in cases of tottering and painful weakness.

The

which must necessarily fan, not damp, the morbid flame; but when the inflammatory temperature is much reduced, and verging on extinction from the effect of topical cold, narcotic virtue may then operate beneficially in calming, both locally and generally, the irritative and sentient commotion which the violence of pain had induced.

The morbid irritability which arises from systematic weakness or atony consequent on the debilitating effect of protracted gout, is the peculiar condition which requires the energizing and quieting influence of opiate and narcotic power.

No dose of opium compatible with human existence, will alleviate the extreme torture of

The immoderate operation of opium, as well as that of every other narcotic substance, may indirectly induce eventual debility, by the exhausting effect of undue excitement; but this will, in common with other instances of deficient motive energy, be characterized by a small, unequal, and rapid action of vital power, and not by augmented tone and slowness. It may be justly concluded therefore, that opium, and all other narcotic agents, are impressively and diffusively stimulant, capable of universally pervading the system, and of annulling the irregular and rapid actions of trembling atony, by equalizing and energizing the motions of vital power.

gout.

gout. When given in this disease with unrestrained freedom, it induces ferocious delirium, which is followed by an aggravated sense of local pain. Thus it appears, that the only remedy for gouty inflammation is that which a law of nature has marked out, as peculiarly adapted to the cure of the disease, consisting of the most prompt method of extinguishing fire. This is more or less effected by any cold medium, but most commodiously, and in general very efficaciously, by water at the atmospheric temperature.

It is redundant heat only that is the object of removal in gouty excitement; that which is natualr is organized, forming the very principle of life itself, therefore cannot offend, and could not be transferred without partial decomposition, disease, and death; but that which distemper generates is uncombined, and will inflame and destroy the parts on which it is evolved, if suffered to amass, and not early evaporated or diffused through media at a lower temperature.

In every attempt to reduce distempered heat, intestinal obstruction should be obviated as a source of visceral pressure and systematic irritation. An occasional laxative therefore should

be

be given, to remove costiveness in gouty affection, and to prevent its morbid consequences.

It is not necessary to reduce the systematic
strength by evacuation, in the cure of gout : this
would be to superadd constitutional weakness
to the local inflammation, farther to disturb the
general health, to incur more severe sympathetic grievances, and to retard the progress of
convalescence. The disease is local ; the constitutional strength, then, should neither be inordinately stimulated, nor broken, but preserved
as unimpaired as the painful conflict will admit.

Neither bleeding nor purging therefore is
indicated in the cure of gout. Abstinence
from fermented liquors, drinking cold water as
an ordinary diluent, avoiding salted provisions,
and diminishing the accustomed proportion of
animal food, are the only changes in the usual
diet, which the most speedy cure of gout would
appear to require.

4. The view which has been here taken of
gouty disease, clearly exhibits the incongruity of
attempting its relief, by the accustomed mode
of increasing the local temperature.

If

If the excitement already is so violent, as to have induced the most exquisite pain, and to have endangered the production of altered struc- ture, surely the stimulant influence of additional heat must exasperate the mischief, and render the affection truly deplorable.

It is much to be lamented, that the investi- gation of disease is thought to be the exclusive province of abstraction, and that science can only be cultivated by intellectual refinement, soaring above the reach of common sense.

To this disregard of the evidence of feeling must be ascribed the preposterous practice of endeavouring to cure gout by aggravating its violence, and protracting its duration.   Common sense is shocked at the absurdity; but the pride, the dogmatism, and perverseness of notional science, imagine a justification for the error, and prohibit the exercise of a rational opinion on the subject.   Increased temperature in gouty affection, whether proceeding from systematic or local warmth, must necessarily lay the found- ation of the worst effects, and does really occasion the irreparable, and often horrible ravages, which occur on the affected parts.   It is the fostered continuance of gouty excitement

3   in

in the ligamentous and tendinous structure, that induces decomposition of fabric, and reduces joints but simply inflamed, to the unsightly wreck of tophous or shapeless tumefactions, grievously torn by the deposition, concretion, and exclusion of calcareous matter. These are among the effects of mismanaged and protracted gout, the aggravated mischief of erroneous treatment, unknown to the unexasperated course of inflammation, the mighty work of science, and the disgrace of common sense.

It may be truly said, that the gouty deformities which so often present, are not the necessary or unavoidable consequences of the disease, but the lamentable effects of artificially stationing morbid excitement, on parts which cannot endure protracted inflammation, without incurring irretrievable damage.

The truth of this fact may be familiarly illustrated by what occurs in mismanaged inflammation on any other structure than that of the ligamentous and tendinous. It is invariably found, that increased heat topically applied to the inflamed part, by either poultice or fomentation, progressively augments the stimulus of vascular distention, until at length, either from

mechanical

mechanical violence, or the repulsive force of accumulated heat, the fabric begins to demolish, the
organic affinities by which the constituent principles of the diseased parts were connected, yield,
and injury beyond regeneration is sustained.
That equal mischief should occur in a texture
that admits not of the slightest deviation, consistently with the due execution of its office, is
too evident to be insisted on.

The local evils of the protracted gout do not
fill the measure of injury produced by its continuance. The morbid sympathies which the
habitual pain generates in the system, become
at length highly irritable, and may be awakened
into serious affections, by the various remote
causes of disease: this is often so much the
case, that the gouty system becomes a most
impressible thermometer, as well as barometer,
to all considerable changes in aerial temperature,
and density.

Is it no reflection then on art, to have
fettered nature in inextricable disease, and, under
the semblance of a remedy, to have consolidated
the worst conditions of both general and local
distemper?

It

It has been seen that gouty inflammation requires the reverse treatment to that which is
commonly employed; that the redundant heat
should be transferred by cold media, with all
possible dispatch, which would prevent the
effects resulting from stimulant influence, and
which so often torture, cripple, and disfigure
its unhappy victims.

There are indeed two modes of reducing inflammatory heat: the one is by diffusion, or
transference through substances at a lower temperature; the other is by exhausting the fuel,
or the pabulum which evolves it: thus, combustive force will diminish, as the final destruction of the burning body approaches; but it
must be remembered also, that it will cease
altogether, when the body is wholly burnt:
in like manner organic structure may be so stimulated, as at length to be nearly exhausted of
vital power, and consequently be reduced to
languid motion; but here too, its total exhaustion is hazarded, which would be tantamount
to death itself. No difficulty can occur in
making an election between these two modes of
reducing heat: in that by abstraction, life is
shielded against the destructive conflict of combustive agitation; while in that by addition, it

H   is

is exposed to its deranging violence. The one is the direct debility of abstinence; the other, the indirect debility of intemperance.

The seeming contrast which is presented in the cure of inflammatory affection, by cooling and heating, or by anti-stimulant and stimulant powers, may be reconciled, by the attempt to effect a reduction of vital power by opposite means: but who can hesitate a moment to prefer the direct to the indirect method, when the one is immediate, safe, and always practicable, while the other is slow, precarious, and often unattainable?

It is on this crooked principle, that scalds and burns are attempted to be remedied by exposure to fire, and the application of spirit of turpentine; that sprains are treated with stimulant applications; that recent incisions, and contusions, are washed with spirituous embrocations; and that gangrenous inflammation is subjected to the excitant impression of effervescing and fermentative poultices.

This is at best endeavouring to obtain with fire and sword, what may be acquired by peaceful surrender.

5. The

5. The misconceived notion of the constitutional and critical nature of gout, precludes the exercise of common discernment as to its true character, and consigns it to the dominion of the most inveterate prejudices.

The influence of habitual adoption and intellectual indolence, rejects and disdains farther inquiry into a disease that is supposed to be sufficiently understood, and of an accredited nature, that has been consecrated by the concurrent testimony of ages.

Truth has not a more arduous obstacle to contend with, than prescriptive error. It is an authority which is held unquestionable; and though its ground be not understood, it is considered as cavilling or captious, to disbelieve, or doubt, what has been confirmed by unobjected admission.

These impositions can only be detected by an ardent love and desire of independent inquiry, by an aversion to conclusions that neither illustrate any difficulty, nor lead to any advantage.

A guarded endeavour at investigation, in such circumstances of blind fidelity, unmeaning con-

fidence,

fidence, and useless prescription, may terminate in valuable discovery; it will certainly break the fetters of prejudice, and afford an unconfined sphere for liberal contemplation.

The painful severity of gout, its crippling tendency, its deep and irreparable impression on the constitutional strength, and the increasing facility and frequency of its recurrence, are well adapted to impress a belief of the dreadful nature of the malady, and to induce an anxious endeavour to investigate the cause, and to devise a rational mode of repressing and curing so growing and crying an evil. Some diseases are more untractable than others, and some are absolutely incurable; but it is peculiar to gouty inflammation to proscribe every attempt to cure, lest its remedial efficacy should be fatally counteracted.

Such nonsense is sounding, but must vanish before the decree of reason and fact, which here proclaims gout, in common with every other disease, to be fair game for medical attack; that it possesses neither salutary nor morbid privilege; that no quarter should be given to it; but that it should always be earnestly combatted, in a manner a manner commensurate with its speedy and utter extinction.

6. The practicability, as well as urgent necessity, for curing gouty inflammation, must be apparent, from the remarks which have been offered on the nature and tendency of its proximate cause. When the more active violence of the malady has been repressed, and a congenial as well as tolerable temperature may be returning to the affected parts, some attention will be necessary to conduct the convalescent progress, with both local and constitutional advantage.

As soon as the distempered sensibility of the inflamed parts is sufficiently subdued to admit of the pressure of friction, the useful aid of that topical exertion to the debilitated vessels should not be omitted; it should be performed at least three or four times a day, during ten or fifteen minutes at each time, adapting its force exactly to what may be endured without giving pain. Co-operatively with this intention of expediting recovery, the aggrieved parts should be also subjected to voluntary motion, as often and as durably as may be done without occasioning hurtful irritation.

The

The impaired energy of vital power, consequent on inflammatory violence, is much retrieved by the active excitement imparted to the languid state by gentle friction and voluntary motion. They tend also to reinstate the salutary temperature, or active conditions of healthful repulsive motion.

Pursuant to this principle of affording benefit, the affected parts should be kept warmer than is proper, during the active stage of the complaint, and strict bandage may be likewise advantageously applied to the whole limb which may have been the seat of the disease, with a view to the compressive, sustaining, and consequently tonic influence rendered by it.

If uncongenial heat should at any period of convalescence disturb the ease or natural sensation, the bandage should be either wetted previously to its application, in cold water, or be occasionally moistened with that fluid, while remaining on the part.

If an unyielding sense of torpor, weight, and deficient heat should supervene, it should be subdued by bathing at least twice a day, during one hour at each time, the affected part in

warm

warm water, at the temperature of one hundred degrees of Fahrenheit's thermometer, or as hot as the sentient state of the part will admit *.

Violent attacks, as well as the protracted duration of gouty excitement, often deeply undermine the constitutional strength, and expose the general health to the various risks of morbid excitability.

* It is not unusual for the ligaments and tendons, after repeatedly suffering from inflammatory or gouty affection, to become so thickened and indurated, as to give to the diseased joints both an unsightly enlargement, and great difficulty of motion. On these occasions, nothing will more efficaciously contribute to restore to the stiffened joints the lost power of easy flexion, than rubbing them at least three times a day, during half an hour, with mild oily substances, heated to the temperature of the skin. The friction, or rubbing, is best performed with the hand, and its briskness should be so proportioned to the sensation of the part, as never to excite a painful degree of heat. Either the animal oil called neat's-foot oil, or olive oil, is very proper for this purpose; or what indeed is equal, if not superior to either of these, is an aqueous solution of the yolks of egg, prepared by dissolving three yolks of egg in one pint of water. This mode of remedy should be pursued until the desired effect be obtained, which commonly happens in the course of a few weeks, but which may not in very inveterate cases be fully produced in less than two or three months.

This

This is also an obstacle to the local recovery of tonic and native firmness; it should therefore be encountered by the most appropriate means of reinstating systematic energy. This must be attempted by a well-conducted plan of nutriment, taking but a small quantity at a time, at short intervals, slow mastication, and moderate dilution. The diet should consist chiefly of animal food, and, if digestion be much impaired, a small portion of either Madeira or sound Port wine may be permitted.

Dyspeptic oppression may be somewhat remedied by friction, with a flesh-brush, over the region of the stomach; but it will in general, in the most fallen state of digestive power, be effectually obviated by the practical rule of neither taking at once, more than the bulk of half an ounce of any solid substance, nor than three ounces of liquid, at distances of one hour. This regulation is indeed of so much importance, in all cases of convalescence, whether from gouty or any other disorder, that to its rigid observance may be justly ascribed, not only the celerity, but the regularity and ultimate perfection of recovery.

If

If much constitutional debility, irritability, and nocturnal watching should prevail, the peruvian bark, quassia, gentian, and other kindred stomachic tonics, may be employed, and at night the soothing influence of an opiate should not be omitted. Costiveness should be avoided; and air and exercise should be enjoined, as holding a high rank in the scale of tonic power.

It is not to be forgotten in this work of re-trieving constitutional strength, that the suitable means should be uniformly, not desultorily pur-sued, as lost power is not recoverable by pa-roxysmal regularity, but by systematic precision only. The period of convalescence is fraught with anxiety. Emersion from disease is not complete emancipation : though health be in front, distemper is closely in the rear; no secure station presents between them ; a want of salutary progress always endangers a mortal regress. *Non progredi, est regredi.*

Whatever proficiency be made in the cure of gouty excitement, the advantage gained should be incessantly furthered, to obviate relapse, which is a renovation of the disease, under the

aggravated

aggravated circumstances of impaired vital energy and distempered susceptibility for morbid impression. If, however, relapses should occur, the disease will resume its wonted character; it may indeed prove more violent, and less yielding, but in essential principle it will be identically the same. The mode of cure, therefore, should be that which is recommended in the original affection, adapting the force of the remedy to the exigencies of exasperated difficulties; and unremittedly employing it, until a salutary termination be effected.

The mode of curing gout here submitted to public consideration, is not offered as infallible: such a pretension would betray an ignorance of the incurable nature of the disease, when founded in altered and irreparable structure.

This irremediable state has uniformly resulted from neglect and mismanagement, permitting irretrievable injury to be done to the inflamed parts. It may be affirmed without fear of contradiction, that no instance of gouty affection would ever attain an immoveable fixation, by irreparably damaging the ligamentous and tendinous structure, if seasonably and duly treated by reduced temperature. Those therefore who

are

are but in the novitiate of the disease, who are not yet the veteran sufferers characterized by distorted and motionless joints, may be assured that the proposed remedy will prove to them *invariably radical*; and for the consolation of those who bear about the incurable badge of fostered or neglected disease, be it known, that the afflicting pain of renewed attacks will *speedily yield* to diminished heat, will exempt the constitution from the exhausting effect of protracted irritation, and tend greatly to lengthen the intervals of recurrence, though an insuperable obstacle should exist in the altered structure of the diseased parts, to an effectual or permanent cure.

No case of gout then can occur, in which either *curative* or *beneficial* efficacy is not promptly derivable from reduced temperature. In this estimate of its worth, it is entitled to an incomparable preference to any medicinal mode of relief, which either has, or probably ever will be proposed for this grievous malady.

The boasted medicines which have been at times palmed on the public for infallible remedies in this disease, have been a palpable imposition,

sition, a gross abuse of erroneous prejudice and thoughtless credulity. Gout is a disease of redundant temperature, which cannot be controlled by the effect of any medicine operating either generally or locally. Whatever causes a positive excitement must injuriously increase the excessive temperature; and whatever induces no degree of excitement must be wholly inefficient, and of course useless.

Evacuations by bleeding and purging, assisted by slender diet, may tend to relieve; but the effect will not be sufficiently concentrated on the affected parts, to annul the morbid heat. Such an evacuant attempt at cure would also unnecessarily and noxiously impair the systematic energy, protract the period of convalescence, and at best substitute a precarious and complicated mode of remedy, for one that is simple and uniformly efficacious.

Without the gift of prophecy, or hazarding too much to prediction, the laws of the animal economy, as well as the established axioms of medicinal efficiency, warrant the opinion, that no substance, of whatever combination or properties, will ever be discovered, capable of exciting either

either a directly curative, or even palliative influence, on gouty or ligamentous and tendinous inflammation, independently of the aid of reduced heat; or, in other words, that this salutary effect will never be produced by any agent, so appropriately and extensively, as by the topical affusion, showering, or other modes of incessantly applying water, at its prevailing degree of coldness, assisted by cool apartments, abstinence from fermented liquors, dietetic stimulants, and copiously diluting with aqueous and other slender fluids, at the atmospheric temperature.

SECTION

SECTION V.

PREVENTION OF GOUT.

1. THE art of preventing justly claims a precedency to that of curing diseases; and as the power for effecting this desirable object generally exists, the vast catalogue of distempers afflicting human health may be said to be more the result of voluntary errors, than of inevitable necessity.

To no disease does the truth of this remark more forcibly apply than to that of gouty excitement, in all its local forms and systematic sympathies. As life is the effect of stimulant power, and health the result of its due application, it is obvious that indifference to the adjustment of this salutary standard of excitant agency must be attended with frequent deviation and proportionate disease.

Dietetic regulation then is of the utmost importance, in both affording and protecting the salutary conditions of life. It is from the alimentary source that vital excitement is derived,

and

and from its due use is drawn the most perfect health.

The errors of both excess and defect are correspondently manifested in vital action, which will be shaped and characterized by temperamental susceptibility for morbid impression.

Irregularities in diet are not always followed by early, though generally by ultimate disease. The firmness and force of salutary motions are such as successfully to encounter common and incipient difficulties, thereby preventing health from being the sure victim of every dietetic incaution.

Amidst the vast variety of diseases that molest human nature, and more or less derive their origin from dietetic excess, gouty, or ligamentous and tendinous inflammation stands very conspicuously. Habitual indigestion, stomachic oppression, and intestinal flatulency, sooner or later become the familiar inmates of immoderately indulging in alimentary gratification.

These symptoms are founded on systematic debility, indirectly induced by the excessive stimulation of redundant diet. Debility, whether
induced

induced by the undue abstraction or application of excitement, but more particularly the latter, is a morbid state, dangerously susceptible of the worst forms of disease.

In such a situation, no part of the frame is exempt from the burden of disproportionate violence; and experience has taught, that the ligamentous and tendinous structure, from the various circumstances of density, vascular languor, locomotive excitement, and occasional sprains, is peculiarly liable to become the seat of agitated and inflammatory action, when the systematic energy has been either impaired or disturbed by dietetic excess. The avoidance of an evil is much facilitated by knowing the mode of its hurtful operation. It has been observed then, that stomachic oppression and systematic plenitude greatly disorder the general health; and that, in that commotion, the ligaments and tendons may assume an inflammatory action, and exhibit the true character of gouty disease. The work of prevention, therefore, with respect to diet, consists in habitually imposing a strict restraint on the appetite, in always desisting before a disinclination for eating more shall arise, in masticating slowly and minutely, and in uniformly preserving that unoppressed state of stomach,

mach, and correspondent feeling of systematic health, which invariably attend an unloaded state of that organ, an uninterrupted digestion, and a moderate supply of general nutriment.

To produce this desirable benefit, and to realize its efficacy in preventing gout, an undeviating rule should be observed, of eating but a small quantity at a time. If the appetite might be restrained by weight and measure, the utmost allowance at one meal should not exceed half a pound of solid food, or a pint of liquid. The quality of the nutriment is of less importance than the quantity; in this respect, therefore, the bias of palate may be somewhat indulged. The best diluent for common use, is unquestionably water, though, if the restriction of a pint be observed, the relish may be allowed an equal scope of preference to that conceded to aliment. Cider, beer, wine, and even spirit diluted with water, may be therefore moderately used with impunity, and compatibly with the prevention of gout.

Aliment may be taken under these restrictions two or three times a day; but a late meal, or supper, should be discarded, as unseasonable, oppressive, and of hurtful tendency.

I

, If

If in the general course of health this mode of diet be requisite to obviate the approach of gouty malady, its observance will be additionally necessary when morbid irritations wander over the frame, and threaten to become stationed on the joints: the utter avoidance, at that time, of fermented liquors and animal food would probably crush the evil in its embryon or forming stage, and prevent its evolution.

The abstemiousness here enjoined, may be justly held as a severe infringement on the social ordinances of table freedom; but it must be recollected, that the question is not, whether the pleasurable gratification of the palate should or should not be indulged, but whether the price of frequent gout will be paid for such enjoyment.

The cause of temperance may indeed be safely rested on its own moral and physical merits; but its recommendation acquires irresistible force, by being at once a bulwark against gout and most other forms of disease.

2. Exercise is a genial source of salutary motion in the animal economy. The whole frame is constructed of motive machinery. Vital motion proceeds incessantly and involuntarily; and

that

that which is connected with the larger scale of muscular structure, and subjected to volition, should be moderately exerted in the service of health.

It is impossible that the functions of life can be performed with due energy, unaided by loco-motive excitement.

The universal friction of surfaces, and conse-quent evolution of repulsive or vital motion, oc-curring in bodily exercise, distributes tone and strength over the frame, and balances in due harmony the sentient and irritative actions of the system.

Innumerable are the forms of disease liable to result from inaction. Unwieldy plenitude, un-equal distribution of the circulating fluids, vis-ceral obstructions, vitiated secretions, and dis-tempered excitability, are inseparably connected with a habit of indolent and sedentary in-dulgence.

Gouty excitement, or ligamentous and ten-dinous inflammation, is very likely to arise in this impaired state of health; it is therefore ob-vious that this malady will be powerfully resisted

by

By the effects of such moderate exercise as would conduce to preserve unimpaired the salutary conditions of life.

Diet and exercise mutually depend on each other for their due agency in the animal œconomy. An adequate use of both is indispensable; but the respective sufficiency must in some measure be determined by relative influence.

The mischief of too full a diet may be somewhat countervailed by increased exercise, by which, vital power is more largely expended, and the superfluous load dissipated : on the contrary, abstemiousness does not require equal exertion, as the claim for nutritive supply is proportionately diminished. It is difficult, therefore, to lay down a general rule for the degree of exercise necessary in the prevention of gout. It must depend on constitutional and nutritive circumstances, and be varied as these are more or less powerful and abundant.

The mode of exercise may be also adapted to individual convenience; but, when commodiously practicable, walking is more appropriately suited to oppose the recurrence of gouty malady, than either horse or carriage conveyance. Walking

more

more directly and equably puts the joints in motion than any other mode of exertion, and thus tends more particularly to strengthen the ligamentous and tendinous structure; but it is obvious this good effect is only compatible with moderate walking; too much exertion in that way will induce indirect debility on the ligaments and tendons, or even sprain them; which would tend to produce rather than obviate gout.

Brisk friction, daily performed on those joints that may have already suffered from gouty inflammation, would likewise be proper, for the purpose of concentering the motive exertion on those parts more effectually than could be done by gentle exercise.

The preventive exercise, which is necessary against gout, is that which is pleasurable in common health, and calculated to obviate the oppression, and other ills of nutritive redundancy consequent on habitual inaction.

3. In unequal temperature may be sought a fertile source of disturbed health; and no disorder is more directly in its influence than gouty inflammation. The pernicious operation of irregular heat on the animal economy, arises either

from

from its immediate force, or from the morbid
susceptibility existing in the system to be impressed by its changes. Robust health will endure a range of temperature with impunity, that
would deeply affect an unduly irritable state of
vital power. In the latter description of diseased
excitability are the hurtful effects of variable
temperature to be chiefly expected, though indeed the utmost constitutional strength often
bends its firmness to the mischievous force of
sudden and contrasted changes in the prevailing
temperature. As a common cause of gout,
therefore, variable temperature should engage
the most vigilant precaution against its influence.

The degree of atmospheric heat cannot be so
controlled as fully to obviate the hurtful effects
of its vicissitude. A choice of climate least liable
to deviation from standard warmth is the only
practicable correction of that general evil; but
the most variable temperature from geographical
position may have its noxious tendency resisted,
by sustaining as much as possible an equal degree
of heat on the surface of the body, by avoiding the concentrated heat of fire, of confined
lodging-rooms, and close apartments in the day-
time.

The

The cuticular heat, and with that the due temperature of the whole system, may be preserved with tolerable uniformity, by sheathing or covering the body with flannel. It should be worn next the skin, and its use continued throughout the year, taking it off at going to bed and resuming it on rising.

It is on the surface of the animal body the salutary temperature adjusts and preserves its due balance. Either excessive perspiration, or extreme atmospheric cold, may detach too much heat, while a deficient distribution of the circulating fluids to the skin, arising from various causes of deranged excitability, is attended with diminished perspiration, and consequently an insufficient evaporation of heat. It will then be of the highest importance in preventing gout, as well as various other diseases, to regulate the temperature with the utmost precision, to attain indeed, if possible, a firm inaptitude to easy impression; but guardedly to protect the surface from the injury proceeding from its being exposed to the hurtful conflict of unequal temperature.

Though the heat of the system at large is the first object of regulation, yet that of the joints in particular should not be disregarded.

If

If either excessive or deficient warmth should occur on them, it should be appropriately treated: in the one case, reduced by exposure and cold ablution; in the other, by friction, warm bathing, and temporary increase of covering.

The augmented heat induced throughout the system, and more abundantly on the joints, by excessive exertion, should be suffered gradually to subside, by slow evaporation from the surface, and not be diverted to visceral or other parts, by the effect of sudden cold interrupting the increased distribution or determination of fluids to the skin.

Gouty affection is imminently endangered by every instance of accumulated or disproportioned heat; it should therefore be dissipated with the utmost dispatch, to prevent its becoming stationed, and thereby associatively disturbing the salutary motions of other parts of the system.

The common causes of distempered heat will be effectually avoided by temperate diet, regular and moderate exercise, uniform clothing, and a domestic temperature; at about fifty degrees of Fahrenheit's thermometer.

It

It should be remembered, as a general rule in the conduct of health, that a low temperature is erring on the right side, and more particularly so in repressing and preventing gouty affection.

It is easy to involve the conditions of health in the destructive fury of conflagration; but it is more difficult either to extinguish or derange vital evolution, by depressing or abstracting combustive violence.

4. It should be a leading care in the prevention of gout, to avoid an excessive exertion of the ligaments and tendons, lest a degree of indirect debility should be brought on them, which would be apt to run into inflammatory action on slight occasions, whether general or local. In ordinary exercise even, the joints are exposed to undue violence of motion, which may sprain and induce inflammatory tension. However morbid excitement may be produced on those parts, it should be reduced without delay, to obviate its assuming the gouty character and inveteracy.

It is not even surmised, nor indeed in the prevailing doctrine of gout is it imaginable, that external injury on the ligaments and tendons could

could possibly terminate in gouty inflammation. An entire misconception of the true nature of the disease has led to a total inadvertence to this common source of it.

Though reflection on the disease, through the mists of prejudice, may not suggest the possibility of gout deriving its origin from weakened or sprained ligaments and tendons, yet it is familiar to common observation, that those whose employ subjects them to an extreme use of those parts, such as pedestrian travellers and sportsmen, and particularly the amusive exercise of boys, in jumping, are especially liable to inflammatory affections of the joints. It is also well known, that a part which has been already sprained yields with increased readiness to future exertion, and that frequent relapses impair the motive power of the part, and render it susceptible of being painfully, and often inflammatorily affected by either changes of atmospheric temperature or any derangement of the general health.

The laborious husbandman, whose avocations have connected him with much exposure to inclement weather, and consequently with disturbed distribution of the circulating fluids, feels the

the pressure of ligamentous and tendinous affection with peculiar severity. At one time the affected parts are torpid, stiffened, and deficient in motive energy; at another, redundant heat stimulates them to painful and inflammatory action. But in these circumstances of poverty, temperance, and labour, it would be infringing what is deemed the exclusive privilege of affluence, intemperance, and indolence, to distinguish it by the luxurious epithet *gout*. It nevertheless is really so; and unhappily for the humble sufferer, the refinement of the appellation draws on him the scourge of wealth, without any of its alleviations, by subjecting him to the usual ordinances for the cure of that malady. He is consigned to the routine of increased excitement, and erroneously, though benevolently, furnished with the means of fanning the flame of mischief, to the irretrievable injury of the affected parts.

It must then be admitted, that the earliest dawn of morbid irritation on the ligaments and tendons, whether proceeding from general or local causes, should be assiduously reduced, lest inflammatory action of those parts should announce with *nominal* terror the *real* torture of gouty excitement.

The

The preventive aim of gout, in this way, may be accomplished by temporary inaction of the affected parts, subjecting them to the anti-stimulant or abstracting influence of diminished temperature, by constantly applying to them, during the prevalence of excessive heat, cold water, the avoidance of fermented liquors, somewhat lessening the accustomed quantity of food, keeping the bowels regularly open, occupying a cool and well-ventilated apartment, and preserving a uniform course of mental tranquillity. When all tendency to inflammation has been subdued, the weakened parts should be often rubbed, be kept firmly bandaged, and not be subjected to any stress of exertion, until a due restoration of their motive tone and power shall have been effected.

5. Whatever impairs the energy of vital power has a tendency to induce an unnatural degree of susceptibility for morbid impression generally, and more particularly on the ligaments and tendons, from the disproportionately stimulant effect of locomotive exertion on these parts. Indigestion is in the foreground of noxious influence on the system. It affects the conditions of health radically and universally. While it diminishes the necessary supply of nutriment, it harasses the centre of motive power, by oppressing and

disordering

disordering the stomach, and thus becomes a remote cause of various diseases, and often of gouty affection.

In the endeavour to prevent this disease, the occasional relief, and avoidance of indigestion, should therefore be a principal object of attention. But a moderate quantity of food should be taken at a time, and both slow and minute mastication should be observed. Nothing by way of supper should be taken, and an unoppressed state of the stomach should by exact temperance be steadily preserved.

If indigestion be obviated, a fertile source of other chronic forms of disease will be annulled, which might give an occasion to gouty excitement.

Every variety of affection, whether acute or chronic, febrile, inflammatory, or nervous, may induce gouty disease by distempering the general excitability, and being determined to the ligamentous and tendinous structure: thus it is always difficult to say what modes of disease may lurk in a disordered state of the system, and what may be either their general or local issue.

The

5. The liability to gouty excitement, presenting in the train of every disease, claims, in a preventive view of this malady, the utmost attention to preserving unimpaired the various conditions of general health, by protecting the systematic excitability from morbid impression, either generally or locally. This desirable security is best attainable by rigid temperance, moderate exercise, and equable temperature.

6. The joints of the hands and feet are more particularly liable to gouty affection, from the ligaments and tendons of these parts being especially subject to partial violence, being remote from the vital sources of motive energy, and being much exposed to the pernicious influence of variable temperature.

Occasional flushing, and chilliness of the palms of the hands and soles of the feet, denote the readiness with which these parts lose, either originally or sympathetically, the salutary standard of heat.

To prevent this collective influence from proceeding to the constitution of gout, in addition to the general means already proposed for repressing the formation and obviating the attack

of

of that disease, it would be advisable to wash the feet, as well as hands, every morning at least, in cold water. The tonic effect of this practice will soon be perceived. The muscular, tendinous, and ligamentous parts, in that situation, would derive from it an unyielding degree of healthful strength and firmness. Neither will distempered heat be likely to originate in them, nor to be determined thither from the system by sympathetic or associative connexion.

The temporary reduction of heat by the periodical use of cold water, will at once transfer accidental redundancy of it, and restore the parts to that native energy, in which a due measure of vital power is generated, and in which salutary excitement obtains, undisturbed by morbid agitation.

If a durable sense of chilliness should remain on the part after cold ablution, gentle friction will soon restore the deficient temperature to the healthy standard.

Gouty affection is invited to the extremities, particularly to the feet, by the prevailing practice of clothing them too warmly, from an anxious dread of taking cold, not recollecting that

that cold rarely results from low temperature, but from the inequality in which excessive heat is or can be supported on a part. Cold, therefore, arises from immoderate heat, and would be better described by the phrase of *caballing heat*, than by that of *cold*, which in fact is literally the case.

In advising a part not to be kept unduly warm, it must not be inferred that it should be kept cold; but that the motive power should be left to adjust, in the balance of healthful feeling, the just degree of temperature.

As the sense of either hot or cold is unnatural, the intermediate state, in which neither the one extreme nor the other is discoverable, is that which is healthful, and to the maintenance and recovery of which, a strong innate tendency invariably prevails. It should therefore be an endeavour of art to assist this natural disposition in correcting every morbid deviation, and in duly trimming and equably preserving the just level of salutary temperature.

7. The forming period of gout is sufficiently slow to admit of its progress being repressed, and its completion obviated. To effect this object, both

both the general and local temperature should be assiduously reduced at the earliest appearance of inflammation on the ligamentous and tendinous structure. Instead of the common practice of inviting the disease by increased heat, and other modes of stimulant treatment, the most cooling and unirritating plan of management should be pursued, until every inflammatory symptom shall have fully subsided.

Much unnecessary violence may be prevented by early refrigeration in the incipient stage of gouty malady. If it were suitably resisted before either much local derangement or systematic sympathy shall have rendered a given course of disease inevitable, but little or no real complaint would arise.

A cool apartment, frequent application of cold water to the heated part, diluting plentifully with the same fluid, avoidance of all fermented liquids, a diet so chosen as neither to heat from quality nor oppress from quantity, and an unobstructed state of the bowels, will effectually subdue the rising disease, and remove every obstacle to returning health.

K   SECTION

SECTION VI.

RECAPITULATION.

1. THE earliest records of medicine attest the existence of gouty inflammation.

2. THE frequent occurrence of this malady, in distempered excitability, without any evident cause, either internal or external, has conferred on it the salutary distinction of being curative of other diseases ; it has therefore been uniformly considered, rather as a remedial, than a morbid affection.

3. This erroneous opinion of its nature, and healthful influence, has survived the correction which enlightened reason afforded to the small-pox, the plague, and other forms of inflammatory diseases; in which stimulant treatment, and inviting and protracting the distemper on the surface, were also judged to be the only safe and efficient means of cure ; but which unprejudiced observation ultimately proved to be

fatally

fatally hurtful, and that the very reverse was, the most salutary that could be adopted.

4. The local character of gouty inflammation, and its not so frequently involving the safety of, life, unhappily excluded it from the benefit of analogical explanation and assistance.

5. The nature of gout is purely inflammatory, and possesses no peculiar or specific properties to distinguish it from common inflammation, but what are referable to the structure or organization of the affected parts.

6. The seat of the gout is exclusively in the ligamentous and tendinous fabric; the texture of which, when inflamed, affords all that is peculiar or characteristic of gout. This fabric therefore is necessary to the constitution of what is called gouty inflammation, which evinces that it cannot occur on any of the visceral or vital organs, as these possess nothing of the ligamentous or tendinous structure.

7. The several appellations of gout, rheumatism, and sprain, are only nominally different; they in fact describe identity of affection. Any external variation which may present in the

K 2 degree

degree and progress of the disorder does not
alter the fundamental sameness of the disease,
which consisting in an inflammatory irritation
of the ligamentous and tendinous structure, will
exclusively remain such, however variously and
capriciously denominated.

8. The origin of gout must necessarily be
always local, as it can only arise in inflammatory
affection of the ligaments and tendons, which
are stationed almost exclusively at the joints, and
are not co-extended with the system. The peculiar seat of gouty malady at once chains it to
the ligamentous and tendinous structure, and
gives an undeviating resemblance to its external
character. It necessarily originates in every instance in the same natural circumstances, and
therefore invariably denotes its existence, by the
most unequivocal symptoms.

9. The diffusion, or propagation, of gout, from
the affected joints, is governed by associative or
sympathetic influence of motive power; but
when arrested on any particular organ, as the
brain, stomach, or bowels, it is not characteristic gout in those parts, but simple irritation;
the ligamentous and tendinous structure, necessary to gouty inflammation, being wanting in
those

those vital organs. Nor does the local irritation of gout subside by sympathetic distribution, but in the proportion as the severity of pain may have harassed and exhausted the systematic strength. The consequent general debility will then reduce the local inflammation, and occasion those painfully irregular or agitated motions (usually termed spasm) over the system, which always endanger life, and do often actually terminate in death. Gout therefore cannot be strictly repelled; and when it subsides, and the system becomes affected, it is the consequence of extreme reduction of constitutional strength, by protracted pain, and which might have been prevented by its seasonable relief.

The general health can suffer no other injury from gouty inflammation, than what is occasioned by the debilitating and distempering influence of durable irritation; its early removal therefore renders the disease both mild and safe.

10. The local symptoms of gout are those of common inflammatory excitement, with the only difference of being somewhat modified in the approach and eventual violence, by the peculiar structure of the ligaments and tendons. The

substantial

substantial fabric of those parts is dense, firm, unyielding, and, in its healthy state, comparatively insensible; hence, inflammatory distention of its vascular texture obtains slowly, and without early severity of pain. This is the forming stage of gouty excitement, which serves, sooner or later, to awaken that violent degree of morbid sensibility, which characterizes ligamentous and tendinous inflammation, and arises from the painful conflict occurring between morbid distention and organic resistance. The efforts of the struggle are the local symptoms of gout, consisting of a sense of burning heat, gnawing pain, exquisite sensibility to pressure, tumefaction, efflorescence, shining cuticular distention, and immobility of the affected joint. These appearances will vary in degree of violence, according to the motive condition of the affected parts, but will always sufficiently distinguish the nature of the existing inflammation.

11. The general symptoms of gouty inflammation will depend on the temperamental, habitual, or morbid excitability of the system at large, or of any particular organ. If equal health should pervade the frame, no serious impression need be dreaded; but if distempered excitability

should have fixed its abode on any particular part, the accumulated weight, or concentered force of sympathetic irritation, may so heavily befall it, as to manifest every degree of violence from transient to inflammatory excitement. But whatever be the situation or extent of the morbid impression, its nature will be conformable to the structure and office of the affected part, and not to the character of gouty, or ligamentous and tendinous inflammation.

12. Both the local and general violence of gouty attack must depend on the tone and excitability of the affected parts, and those of the system at large. If resisting or healthful energy should guard the motive powers of the ligaments and tendons, the inflammatory action will be neither violent in its approach, nor obstinate in its duration; on the contrary, should morbid excitability afford a promptness for becoming affected, the onset will be forcible, and its continuance lasting. Similar conditions in the motive powers of the system, will subject them to correspondent affections. If the general strength be firm and unyielding, the local pain will not propagate its influence either systematically or viscerally; but if atony or undue excitability prevail, quick sympathy may either

generally

generally or partially share in the local irritation.

13. The protracted or natural duration of
gout tends to produce irreparable local derangement on the part affected, and a state of the
system promptly susceptible of common causes
of morbid impression. The diseased joints will,
by its long endurance, become contracted, and
be farther distempered by altered structure, by cal-
carcous or osseous, and other vitiated secretions;
while the general motive powers of the system
will be tremblingly alive to every occurring irritation. This deep and complicated mischief is
only to be obviated by an early and radical removal of the disease.

14. The natural or uncurtailed duration of
gout is fraught with severe injury both to the
affected parts, and to the system at large; its
endurance therefore should not be tolerated
longer than the inefficacy of the means employed for its removal may render unavoidable.
Its accession, abstractedly considered, is simple;
its complicated evils are the offspring only of its
continuance. Its protraction can afford no conceivable benefit, while it manifestly tends to
induce irreparable change of structure in the
affected

affected parts, and to agitate the system with a morbid degree of sympathetic irritation; its earliest and most prompt cure, therefore, is at once warranted by science and implored by humanity.

15. Between gouty and other forms of inflammation, no essential difference subsists; the distinction, therefore, designates only a nominal variation, and specifically refers to an inflammatory degree of ligamentous and tendinous excitement.

This is an important fact, as it at once justifies and demands the earliest and most appropriate cure.

16. The various denominations of gout, such as tonic, atonic, retrocedent, erratic, or misplaced, may be reduced to acute and chronic, as best describing the different states of motive energy, as well in the ligamentous and tendinous structure, as in particular vital organs, or in the system at large.

Local and general tone will give an occasion to the acute character, while atony would impart to the affection a less violent, or more chronic form.

form. The organic or systematic participation results from sympathetic or associative influence with the local pain; but this is not gout, but simple irritation. The necessary structure for gouty affection is wanting in the vital organs; the disease therefore can never be justly said to have either retroceded, to have wandered, or to have been misplaced on them. It is as incapable of ranging to a vital part, as the ligaments and tendons themselves are of being transferred thither; though it is capable of generating and diffusing painful, deep, and extensive sympathies over the system.

17. Undue extension of the ligaments and tendons, and also of the tendinous expansion termed fascia, is followed by inflammatory action, which presents a perfect identity with that inflammation denominated gouty, which often occurs on those parts, without any evident external violence. The pain, tumour, efflorescence, and immobility, are precisely similar, and, in fact, are effects flowing from the same physical source of injury. Ligamentous and tendinous extension from mechanical force, may then be truly considered as a frequent remote cause of gout.

The

The ligaments and tendons are much exposed to inflammatory extension from external violence; also from their almost incessant locomotive exertion are peculiarly liable to that undue exhaustion which terminates in an habitual state of indirect debility. These prove fertile sources of gouty excitement; but another remote cause is to be sought in gradual changes of structure, from distempered excitability, embarrassing the vascular transmission, inducing morbid effusions of coagulable lymph, into which new vessels may shoot, which, with other vitiated secretions, establish a prompt susceptibility for inflammatory or gouty impression.

18. However the ligamentous and tendinous structure may have been distempered by frequent inflammation, its nature, tone, or healthful motive energy, will at length undergo so radical a change, as to become an integrant condition of life, capable of generative transmission, or hereditary transference to offspring. This transmittable or intrinsic state of the disease is founded in an innately distempered condition of temperamental excitability, preponderately affecting the ligamentous and tendinous structure; but the disposition only to the disease is here natively furnished, which will not become formally

mally active, without the adequate influence of other noxious powers: thus an hereditary disposition to gout may be kept in motionless abeyance, by withholding from it morbid excitement.

19. Change of temperature, inducing catarrhal affection, by deranging the equable distribution of the circulating fluids, is as common a cause of gouty, as of other forms of inflammatory affection. The morbid excitement which partial plenitude may occasion, in disturbed circulation, from irregular temperature, usually falls on either the membranous, bronchial, or vascular structure of the lungs, inducing catarrhal or peripneumonic disease; but it may also be determined to the ligaments and tendons, and there excite gouty or inflammatory affection. This may occur indeed even originally, but will be more liable to happen when those parts have acquired a distempered susceptibility for morbid impression from former disease.

20. Vascular plenitude, as well as stomachic oppression from immoderately indulging in food, may distemper systematic excitability, and be determined with inflammatory or gouty violence to the ligaments and tendons.

The

The salutary proportion of nutriment bears a strict relation to the exigencies of personal exertion. A sedentary habit of life, and full diet, readily encumber the system with a morbid surcharge of fluids; while active exercise obviates superfluity by motive exhaustion.

In as far as either vascular plenitude or stomachic oppression tends to induce gouty excitement, it may be effectually prevented by an abstemious course of diet, by observing the important practical rules of taking but a small portion of aliment at a time, and of always desisting before the appetite be fully satiated.

21. The stimulant effects arising from an excessive use of fermented liquors, induce a degree of indirect debility, tremulously susceptible of every variety of diseased impression, and, among others, to an inflammatory or gouty excitement of the ligaments and tendons. In this exhausted and agitated state of motive energy, painful irritation may occur on any part; but in no situation will there be tone or energy sufficient to sustain durable inflammation: hence the temperamental atony of intemperate drinkers disfigures and obscures every occurring disease by informality, and want of permanent station.

22.

22. Irregular secretions and excretions, whether of urine, perspirable matter, bile, mucus, habitual piles, or accustomed drains, may induce either general or partial plenitude, vitiate excitability, and prove a remote cause of gouty determination to the ligaments and tendons.

23. Indigestion, imperfect chylification, and habitual costiveness, have conjointly a powerful tendency to vitiate stomachic excitability, to associatively distribute its morbid influence over the system, and (when disproportionate susceptibility for diseased impression exists on the ligaments and tendons) more particularly to determine its force to those parts: thus feeble and lingering attacks of gouty inflammation often occur in circumstances of diminished vital energy, from deficient nutriment and disordered obstruction and excitement of the alimentary canal.

24. In whatever manner the general health may be deranged, the effect may be so partially exerted on the ligamentous and tendinous excitability, as to induce gouty inflammation. The imperceptible manner in which the local excitement approaches in this general state of malady, anxiously obscures its nature, and cordially
welcomes

welcomes its appearances, in the vain, the delusive hope of its remedial efficiency. It announces indeed the arrival of a positive disease with a severity of pain, which at once implores and demands an institution of the most prompt and efficacious mode of cure.

25. Gouty inflammation, like most other diseases, acquires by frequent recurrence a facility of return, which soon becomes habitual. The ordinances of health owe much of their fixation and uniformity to the influence of incessant or uninterrupted continuance; those of disease become similarly radicated by long usage. It is therefore of vast importance in a curative view, that an ailment should not become habitually inveterate, and that the gout should, in every stage of its duration, be circumvented and subdued in the most expeditious and efficacious manner, to obviate its familiar or customary establishment.

26. The proximate cause of gout is the aggregate efficiency of the remote causes, or the disease itself. It is founded in an excess of heat or repulsive motion generated and evolved from simple and compound atomical surfaces: thus perfect identity with respect to the object subsists

subsists between the various denominations, repulsive motion, vital action, and heat. Repulsive motion obtains universally between atoms or corpuscles; vital motion in organic structure; and heat is the impression, or effect, which this repulsive motion makes on the sensorial principle of the animal economy. The excess of heat, then, is the proximate cause of gouty excitement; and consequently its due reduction, its direct, speedy, and effectual cure.

27. Excessive heat has been alleged to be the proximate cause of gout, or to be the disease itself; which obviously suggests as an appropriate indication of cure, an early and unremitted endeavour to allay the morbid temperature on the affected parts, and that the means of reducing it should be proportioned or commensurate to the violence of the disease.

28. Cold water is the universal boon of nature, the common medium of salutary temperature, as derived from the repulsive or motive conditions of the atmosphere; its uniform application, therefore, to parts suffering under gouty inflammation, by either ablution, showering, or immersion, is a remedy as efficacious as simple for that malady. Inveterate cases, or the high temperature

perature of tropical climates, may (though very rarely) require the aid of artificial cold, obtained from a solution of neutral salts in water, effectually to extinguish the inflammatory heat. The application of diminished temperature should be uninterruptedly continued, until the painful sense of heat be reduced. This usually happens within forty-eight hours, almost invariably before the expiration of seventy-two hours. The avoidance of all dietetic, medicinal, and mental excitement, at the same time, would likewise greatly co-operate in the intention of cure.

29. The reduction of the distempered heat, which occasions gouty inflammation, is so readily and completely in the power of cold water, as to preclude the necessity of medicinal assistance. Cases of extreme torture may indeed be somewhat co-operatively soothed by opiate or narcotic influence; but this auxiliary aid will avail nothing, without the incessant application of cold water, and with its employ, will be in general superfluous. Costiveness should be removed, or obviated by occasional laxatives. Neither purging, nor an increase of any other evacuation, is necessary, and by breaking the general strength may prove hurtful.

L

30.

30. The effects of attempting the cure of gout by increased temperature, according to the prevailing practice, are deplorably seen in the ravages this disease is often compelled to make. Disfigured joints, lameness, and systematic, as well as local susceptibility for morbid impression on the slightest occasions, awfully attest the misery which misapprehension of the real nature of the malady entails on its hapless victims, by instituting the most pernicious mode of treatment. Increased temperature never has, nor ever can prove remedial in gout, but by exhausting vital power, to a degree that might induce a state of indirect debility, incapable of sustaining inflammatory action; but this must always be a precarious issue, and is opposed by the certain (perhaps irreparable) mischief, which such superadded violence must necessarily occasion.

By withholding or abstracting heat, its effect is directly prevented. Is not ignition more consistently reduced by diminishing, than by adding, fuel or combustible substances?

31. A correct knowledge only of the real nature and pernicious effects of gout, can remove the inveterate prejudice which contends

for

for its salutary influence, and forbids its speedy and radical cure. It is the only disease that is cherished as possessing remedial powers; nor can it be expected to be treated on any consistently curative plan, while such an erroneous notion is entertained. Undeluded reason, and incontestable fact, authorize its most prompt cure, on the soundest principles of humanity and medical science.

32. The convalescence of gout will require the same attention to further and confirm its progress, as is necessary in that of other violent diseases. A well-conducted plan of nutriment should be regarded as of the first importance in expediting and ensuring perfect recovery. Local friction also, and even topical warm bathing, would be advisable, if an unyielding sense of either torpor or coldness should prevail on the affected part.

Should a relapse actually occur, it should be treated as the original attack, with such adaptations as the circumstances of aggravated or diminished violence may require.

33. Gouty excitement often results from the excessive stimulation of inordinate diet and

fermented

fermented liquors, from intemperately indulging in a larger portion of them than either the stomach can digest, or the system require for salutary nutriment.

. The stomachic oppression, and systematic plenitude, which this alimentary or rather voluptuous abuse occasions, unduly exhausts motive energy, induces indirect debility, and consequently the distempered susceptibility for morbid impression, which is inseparably allied to that agitated and enfeebled state. These hurtful effects, the hot-bed of gouty, and the various other affections of a weakened and vitiated excitability, may be prevented by a rigid avoidance of dietetic excess and an immoderate indulgence in fermented liquors. Small quantities of food at a time, well masticated, and a proportionately limited dilution, with slender fluids, will prove almost certainly preventive of gouty ailment.

34. Habitual exercise, sufficient equally to distribute the circulating fluids, to balance the various secretions, and to obviate nutritive redundancy, will be found importantly conducive to the prevention of gout.

Inactivity

Inactivity is a fruitful source of disease, by withholding the genial excitement of locomotive exertion, and thereby incurring the evils of unwieldy plenitude and distempered excitability, which experience evinces to be peculiarly apt to preponderate on the ligaments and tendons, in the form of gouty inflammation.

35. Gouty, or ligamentous and tendinous inflammation, is not less under the influence of temperature, than that of the various viscera. It should therefore be equalized with the utmost uniformity, that neither its general nor local derangement may be productive of such irregularity in the distribution of the circulating fluids, or in the action of vital power, as may induce inflammatory or gouty ailment.

36. Violent extension of the ligaments and tendons should be avoided, as directly tending to impair their tone, to vitiate their excitability, and consequently to render them easily susceptible of inflammatory affection. When undue violence has occurred on those parts, the earliest sensation of augmented heat should be combated by diminished temperature, applied through the medium of cold water, with which the seat of grievance should be either often washed, or

incessantly

incessantly covered, until the natural sense of warmth shall be restored.

37. An highly irritable state of the system, whether induced by acute or chronic affection, strongly disposes to gouty disease, by rendering the ligaments and tendons more particularly liable to inflammatory excitement, from the disproportionately stimulant effect of locomotive exertion on these parts.

Indigestion, unequal temperature, and habitual inaction, are common causes of this universally morbid impressibility of motive power, which is apt to occasion gouty affection, by preponderating on the ligamentous and tendinous structure.

38. The ligaments and tendons, partly from being distant from the centre of motive energy, and partly from the variable heat to which they are exposed by locomotive exertion, are particularly liable to suffer from unequal temperature and atony. This state may be corrected, and its tendency to gouty affection repressed, by habitually washing every morning at least, the feet, as well as hands, in cold water, briskly wiping them after each ablution, with

with a coarse cloth, for the benefit of friction, until they shall be perfectly dry.

39. Gouty ailment may be either obviated, or arrested in its forming stage, so as to prevent its developement, by resisting the earliest approach of excessive temperature, either generally or locally, by topical cold, aqueous dilution, abstemious diet, cool apartments, avoidance of costiveness, and every other source of morbid excitement, whether universal or partial.

APPENDIX:

CONTAINING

CASES OF GOUT,

&c.

IN WHICH

.THE DOCTRINE LAID DOWN IN THE PRECEDING PAGES
HAS BEEN PRACTICALLY AND SUCCESSFULLY APPLIED;

TO WHICH ARE ADDED

OCCASIONAL NOTES,

DESIGNATED BY THE LETTER K,

BY DR. KINGLAKE.

———————

Longum iter per præcepta; breve, et efficax, per exempla.
SENECA.

INTRODUCTION.

THE preceding doctrine on the nature and cure of gout would be justly held to be much too questionable for implicit admission, if it stood merely on a theoretic basis. On such a ground indeed, it would have been presumptuous to have offered it to the public.

Speculative inquiry is a pleasing gratification to those who possess leisure, and taste, for rational reflection; but the mere product of imagination, unsupported by the evidence of facts, has no claim either to the reputation of science, or to being uttered as practical intelligence. But when adequate trial has ascertained the validity of a theory, it justly challenges acceptance, and will sustain no loss of its intrinsic merit, by either capricious cavilling or unintelligent rejection.

The subsequent Cases therefore are appended to the view which has been here held of gout, to

afford

afford it that support which a subject of so much importance indispensably requires. Some of those cases are original, others have been already published in the Medical and Physical Journal, from whence they have been extracted, and are here incorporated for the purpose of presenting the reader with a collective account of what has hitherto been done, in the refrigerant mode of curing gout.

In justice to neglected experience, it may be affirmed. that many less decisive instances of benefit, than those recited, have been omitted, both to avoid a voluminous Appendix, and the suspicion of having too anxiously pressed the recommendation of the treatment by equivocal testimony.

The evidence offered, is sufficient to warrant a procedure in the practice, which promises ultimately to remove all doubt, and to ensure it a confident and universal adoption.

ROBERT KINGLAKE.

Taunton,
February 1st, 1804.

I. *Dr. Kinglake's first Publication on the Cure of Gout. Extracted from the Medical and Physical Journal, for the Year* 1801.

" To the Editors of the Medical and Physical
Journal.

" Gentlemen,

" Arthritic affections have long been denominated the *opprobria medicorum* ; nor have medical practitioners discovered much solicitude to acquit the healing art of such a degrading charge of incompetency. In no instance of disease has prejudice more arbitrarily usurped the empire of reason, than in the treatment of gout. The crude notion suggested by the humoral pathology of the ancients, that every distemper characterized by cuticular determination, should be considered as originating from some morbid condition of the fluids, requiring specific expulsion from the system, led also to the conclusion, that gout was to be similarly rejected ; hence the routine practice of fostering arthritic inflammation by the topical use of increased temperature, and the internal employ of stimulant medicines, with a view to obviate its retrocession, and to
ensure

ensure its final extinction on the part affected. This procedure has invariably appeared to me to be repugnant to the indication of relief furnished by every constitutional and local feature of the disease.

" Observation and reflection have forced on my conviction the *fact*, that, however loose the analogy might be between the respective proximate causes of ordinary phlegmonous and arthritic inflammations, the resemblance is sufficiently close, in the degree of concomitant temperature. In both, the vascular actions of the system, and of the part affected, generate a morbid excess of heat, alike referable to distempered condition of motive power. Impressed then with the persuasion, that, with regard both to inordinate temperature, and to its general as well as topical manifestation, a radical similitude subsists between these *nominally* different inflammations, it appeared to me strictly warrantable to institute a perfectly similar plan of cure: the event has fully verified its probable utility, as will be evinced in the detail of the subsequent cases.

" A young man about twenty-five years of age, of an healthy temperament, and without any known hereditary predisposition to arthritic affection,

tion, had been during three or four preceding
years attacked at least once, sometimes twice,
in the course of twelve months, with a severe
fit of the gout: it usually affected the great toe
of one foot only; occasionally also both knees,
and one or more of the finger-joints. On these
several parts were permanent inflammation and
tumefaction, arthritically characterized by the
usual shining aspect, and exquisite sensibility to
either touch or motion; morbidly associated
irritation also arose in different parts of the
system, but did not become so concentrated, as to
be either durable or seriously violent.

" The medical advice given to the patient on
those occasions, by different practitioners, was
to consider the complaint as a violent degree of
gout, to cover the affected parts with flannel, to
sustain the powers of life by the occasional use
of stimulants, and resignedly to await the ordinary solution of the disease. This not less
hackneyed than pernicious admonition had been
repeatedly complied with, at the expense of
several months painful durance, and the consequent loss of much constitutional strength. In
the attack preceding the last, after several weeks
confinement, and the injurious effects of high
temperature, my advice was desired. The ligaments.

ments of the great toe joints of one foot, of
both knees, and the wrist of one hand, were at
that time much inflamed, thickened, and swollen, extremely painful on the slightest pressure
or effort at motion; morbidly sympathetic irritation had also pervaded the system, and been
more or less permanently arrested, and evolved
in relative symptoms on the brain, stomach, and
bowels; constitutional atony likewise advanced
to an alarming height, and distempered irritability prevailed in a threatening degree.

" Under these several unfavourable circumstances, no time was to be lost ; much mischief
had already been incurred, by awaiting a natural termination of the disease.

" The local inflammation and irritation appearing to be the chief sources of the evil, it
seemed highly expedient to subdue what in
my estimation constitutes the efficient cause of
these active symptoms, *namely, excessive temperature*; this can only be indirectly accomplished
by reduced heat; and no vehicle is so suitable
to effectuate it as cold water.

" In opposition then to every prejudice, equal
parts of cold water and acetated water of ammonia

monia (aqua ammoniæ acetata *) were directed
to be constantly applied to the affected parts
by means of cloths wetted in that fluid, renewing them every half hour, or even at shorter intervals, if any sense of morbid heat sooner
returned. With this external remedy was combined the internal exhibition of camphorated
tincture of opium (tinctura opii camphorata),
and the ammoniated tincture of guaiacum
(tinctura guaïaci ammoniata), in doses of two
drachms each, repeated every eight hours. The
relief obtained from the topical application of
cold to the parts affected was immediate. The
efflorescence, swelling, and stiffness, were so
far diminished within twelve hours, as to admit
of moderate pressure, and even voluntary motion of the affected joints, with but little inconvenience. The co-operative influence of the
internal medicine seemed to calm the agitated
state of the system, and to dispose to sleep; but
it manifestly, at the commencement, had no

* " My motive for conjoining the acetated water of ammonia
(aqua ammoniæ acetata) with common water, was not with a
view to any discutient quality, which might be supposed to
result from the mixture, but merely to avoid exciting any dread
in the apothecary who furnished it, against the use of cold
water alone, which would have probably proved an impediment
to its due application. "

M   sensible

sensible effect on the local irritation; for, on the third and fourth days, if, as sometimes happened, the application of the cold water was not duly pursued, though the medicine was regularly exhibited, a painful sense of heat, and renovated tension, promptly returned.

" After five days prosecution of this treatment four distinct sources of local irritation were annulled; the system became recruited, and pervaded by an equal distribution of improving vital energy; the appetite returned, digestion amended, and the nights were no longer sleepless. This convalescent procedure happily terminated, in the course of one month, in the full reinstatement of health.

" After an interval of nine months perfect freedom from every symptom of arthritic affection, this patient suffered a renewed attack ; the same parts were preponderately affected with gouty irritation, as in the former instance, but with additional violence.

" It had prevailed upwards of a fortnight before my advice was taken, during which period, the ordinary medicinal treatment in those cases (and
which

which has been already mentioned) was employed, and with the same unavailing effect and deleterious consequence. The disorder became hourly exasperated; every symptom, particularly those of excessive temperature and exquisite sensibility, had been much exacerbated, and ligamentous thickening and inaction had induced absolute inability to move the affected joints without assistance.

"The experience of the past had been too unequivocally demonstrative of the beneficial influence arising from the topical application of reduced temperature, not to be again resorted to. The plan of treatment before recited, was renewed, and with precisely similar effects. In the course of three days, the topical use of the cold fluid had so diminished the local swelling and irritation, as to unfetter the confined joints, and to restore the power of tolerable loco-motion. The medicine before employed was also resumed, with the evident advantage of calming the irregular action of the system, by equalizing the circulation of the vascular fluids, and thereby reinstating the cuticular, and every other disturbed secretion.

" In

" In the course of three weeks, convalescence was so far advanced, as to leave nothing more to complete the cure, than the restoration of natural tone to the debilitated constitution. At this time, now upwards of two months from the date of the attack, this final benefit has been fully accomplished by the conjoint aid of bark, exercise, and a well-regulated course of nutritive diet.

" The most sceptical must admit, that the highly salutary effects of diminished temperature, in this case, are beyond all controversy. In both instances, the neglect of it had permitted the disease to go to an unpromising length; neither natural effort, nor superadded assistance, seemed competent to effect the change necessary to subdue the inflammatory and decomposing process of arthritic irritation. Morbid afflux of fluids on the affected ligaments, had caused the generation of new vessels, which were in turn engaged in carrying on diseased secretion and accretion. Reduced temperature abstracted this distempered action, and, by thus depriving the disordered parts of nutritive supply, exposed them to be spontaneously decomposed, and borne

away

away by exhalant impulse and lymphatic transmission *.

" The value of the evidence afforded by this
case is also much enhanced by its embracing
two instances, in which the curative influence
of reduced heat in arthritic malady was equally
strongly marked. Had the issue however been
somewhat different, it might have been owing
to that perpetual and inscrutable diversity in
temperamental susceptibility, which perplexes
and defeats every endeavour at discovering
any thing like uniformity in the effect of
agents on the animal economy; but the exact-
ness of the coincidence appears to warrant the
important conclusion, that reduced temperature
is capable of such an absolute degree of efficiency
as cannot be either resisted or modified by slight
organic dissimilarity.

" The second subject of topical refrigeration,
under my direction, in arthritic disease, was a

---

* " The phrase lymphatic transmission is here substituted
for the ordinary term *absorption*, it being my opinion that the
lymphatic vessels do not, in any instance, *actively absorb*, but
passively admit the redundant exhalant, interstitial, or extrava-
sated fluids forced into their *permanently open orifices* by arterial
and muscular impulse."

woman

woman aged forty, of an healthy temperament,
who had been grievously tortured upwards of four
months by gouty irritation, inveterately stationed
on the articular ligaments of both ankles, one knee,
and both wrists ; neither of the toes was affected,
nor had the patient, prior to this time, experienced any similar complaint ; yet the peculiarly
glossy tumefaction, efflorescence, and exquisite
sensibility of the affected parts were eminently
characteristic of arthritic disease.   Subordinate
degrees of irritation occasionally wandered over
the system, with the seeming effect of affording
temporary alleviation to the more fixed pain, but
without exonerating the diseased ligaments of
their cumbrous inflammatory load ; indeed the
relief appeared to consist rather in somewhat
diverting the attention from the accustomed
source of grievance, than in its real diminution.
The patient had unsuccessfully tried the probable modes of assistance which reputable
medical advice, during several months, could
afford ; at length, wearied and discouraged by
the fruitless effect of every endeavour, and having
been informed of the benefit which had been
rendered, under my direction, to the patient
whose two cases have been just stated, my
opinion was desired on her situation. It appeared to me at first sight, to be so clearly a

                                                    case

case of morbid temperature; habitually fixed by long standing, and bearing so close an analogy to the preceding cases, that a similar treatment was instituted for her relief, with particular attention to the improvement of her digestion, which indeed had been so much impaired, as to have greatly curtailed the due alimentary resources of vital sustenance. The topical application of cloths wetted in the cold mixture before mentioned, afforded speedy benefit, and its frequent renewal soon restored motive power to the stiffened and disabled joints. With the subsidence of the swellings ceased also the morbid irritation that had reduced the natural energy of the system to a wretched state of atony; hence the powers of life were no longer squandered in diseased motions, but recruited by the renewal of healthy action.

" Three weeks procedure in this mode of resisting local irritation by topically allaying redundant heat, had effected unexpected changes; at the end of one month, a message from the patient desired that something strengthening might be directed, observing, that the swellings and pain were wholly removed, that the disabled joints had regained the power of voluntary motion, and that a retrieval of strength seemed

to be alone wanting to complete the cure : since
that time, now upwards of two months,
no intelligence has reached me concerning the
patient, which induces me to presume on at
least a *satisfactory*, if not a *perfect* recovery.

" This case affords an instructive instance,
that, whatever may be the degree of prevailing
debility, the existence of morbid excess of temperature, whether local in the character of
inflammatory affection, or general in the shape
of febrile irritation, might be safely combated
with rapid and persevering reduction. The debility here present, was incessantly advancing
by the inordinately stimulant effect of the attendant irritation, and would have soon gone to
the extent of fatal exhaustion, had it not been
obviated by the appeasing and regenerating influence of diminished heat.

" The fourth case of this description which
you are requested to indulge me in citing, is
that of a young man much addicted to intemperate drinking, who had been formerly subject,
at irregular intervals, to gouty affection, on the
great toe of one foot only. In the last attack,
my advice was taken on account of an efflores-
cent discolouration diffused over the whole
foot.

foot. This additional appearance to the usual more confined aspect of gout, had induced much alarm for imaginary consequences.

" The arthritic inflammation originated on the second joint of the great toe, was productive of insufferable pain, and consequently of severe symptoms of systematic irritation.

" My former experience of the salutary effects of reduced temperature, emboldened me to confide the welfare of this patient to its *solitary* influence. He was supplied with a pint bottle of cold water (coloured for the purpose of disguise), in which he was directed to moisten a folded cloth, and to envelope with it the whole foot, renewing it as soon as the sense of imparted coldness should be overcome by that of returning heat: this, on an average, was about once in half an hour. The relief obtained was immediate; in a few hours the affected joint could be voluntarily moved; by the following day the cuticular redness over the foot assumed a slightly livid hue, the tumefaction also diminished, and in the course of one week the patient walked about with tolerable convenience. No medicine was directed; abstinence only from immoderate indulgence in spirituous and fermented liquors

was

was enjoined. A tight bandage commencing at the affected toe, and spirally continued over the foot and ankle to the knee, restored in a few weeks the accustomed tone to the enfeebled extremity: thus the strict *podagral* character of arthritic affection was arrested in its progress, and salutarily terminated with unprecedented rapidity by the aid of diminished heat. This case presents an example of unmingled gout safely and expeditiously subdued by the sole external use of cold water. Not the slightest unfavourable symptom arose in the train of its removal; on the contrary, the systematic irritation which appeared to have been excited, and sustained solely by the local pain, ended with the cessation of its cause; and every relick of morbid feeling, whether from habitual or atonic influence, speedily yielded to the renovated conditions of perfect health.

" My observation of the benefit resulting from the topical application of reduced heat in arthritic inflammation, has yet been limited to the four preceding cases. Some indeed who have been veterans in the disorder, and who, from having been prejudiced with the popular notion that its periodical return, and due local support, were essentially necessary to health, could

could not be prevailed on to apply cold water, have yet, on my recommendation, so far relaxed from employing high temperature, as to disrobe the affected parts of flannel, and expose them to the ordinary heat of the atmosphere: the consequence of this partial compliance has been such relief, as to induce a perseverance in the too restricted remedy.

" From what has been related, it appears allowable to infer, that high temperature, whether the cause or effect of the morbid conditions of vital power, which proximately constitute gout, is safely and speedily controllable by the simple application of cold water; that the prevailing opinion relative to the critical nature of that disease on the extremities, is liable to much distrust; that the local deposit is not, as commonly supposed, a particular preponderance and detention of the constitutional disorder, but that it *originates* in the *parts themselves*, and is thence distributed, by associated influence, over the system; that the longer the local affection endures, the greater probability there will be of morbid sympathies being generated, and established on the vital organs, which may terminate in rapid and painful death.

" If

" If these inferences be admitted, the salutary effects of early and incessant low temperature, recited in the preceding cases, will be easily explicable; and it will follow that the true indication of cure in arthritic inflammation will consist in transferring, by cold media, the redundant heat of the part affected.

" It may be demanded, if this refrigerant mode of topically abstracting the stimulus of heat is so efficacious, would not a general antiphlogistic plan, as it is termed, powerfully co-operate in subduing the morbid state of the parts? My observation enables me to answer this question, by affirming, that such collateral aid is not necessary, without warranting me in saying it would be pernicious; but it is rational to expect, that it would be of hurtful tendency by adding to the prevailing systematic debility, and thereby incurring the inseparable danger attendant on extreme weakness and irritability. The salutary influence of topical cold on inflamed surfaces, does not depend on debilitating motive power, but on removing the immoderate excitement which always deranges, and threatens by progressive exhaustion, the ultimate extinction of life: thus the tonic and invigorating effect of affusion with cold water, in febrile affection,

and

and of somenuaii in various chronic diseases, may be explained.

" The most salutary mode perhaps of restoring strength in highly enfeebled and irritable states of motive power, is to abstract all unnecessary, and particularly *painful* excitement. The occasional exclusion of light, avoidance of sound, undue heat, redundant aliment, intestinal constipation, and mental anxiety, will often be found conjointly to promote the regeneration of a greater degree of systematic energy, in default of that power, than could be effected by the best managed employ of medicinal stimulants.

" I am, &c.

" *Chilton super Polden,* " ROBERT KINGLAKE. "
 October 12, 1801.

II. *Dr. Kinglake's second Publication on the Cure of Gout, with an Address to his medical Brethren. —Extracted from the Medical and Physical Journal for the Year* 1803.

" To the Editors of the Medical and Physical Journal.

 " Gentlemen,

" When I last addressed the public through the medium of your Journal, on the salutary

effects

effects resulting from the topical application of
cold water in gouty affection, the practice was
new in my experience; and (as was observed in
that paper) a theoretical view of the analogy
subsisting between gouty and every other description of inflammation, led me to make trial
of its powers. Although popular prejudice
against the mode of remedy is too inveterate to
admit of so extensive an application of it, as is
necessary to bring it into vogue; yet particular
instances have lately occurred in my practice,
which confirm very satisfactorily my former
opinion of its superior curative power.

" Amidst a variety of cases, in which the
topical reduction of temperature rendered much
temporary alleviation, but in which a distrust in
its safety too much interrupted its use, to afford
any decisive testimony on the subject, are the
subsequent examples of its salutary efficiency,
in which its employ was conducted in a manner
that warrants placing the results on the records
of medical facts.

CASE I.

" A gentleman who had repeatedly suffered
under severe paroxysms of gout, experienced,
a few months since, a recurrence of the affection.

It

It shewed itself as usual on the ball of the great toe, which was much swollen, highly inflamed, and exquisitely painful. The local disease soon extended its stimulant influence over the system, inducing violent symptoms of general irritation. The topical inflammation proceeded in the accustomed manner during about a fortnight, when my advice was desired.

" On inquiry, it appeared that the routine treatment of covering the affected part with flannel, had been sedulously observed; confinement to bed in a warm room, and a liberal use of spirituous liquors, were also judged expedient, to obviate every risk of repulsion. By this course the patient had added to the local establishment of the disease, considerable constitutional debility. No circumstance however in the case gave me the smallest concern for the safety of employing very freely reduced temperature, which was applied by means of cloths wetted in an aqueous fluid. This was directed to be repeated every half hour, or even oftener, if a painful degree of heat should sooner prevail. Sudorific medicine composed of camphorated tincture of opium (tinctura opii camphorata), and ammoniated tincture of guaiacum (tinctura guaiaci ammoniata), in doses of two drachms each, diluted with water, was likewise ordered to be taken at intervals of

I

six

six hours. Instantaneous ease arose from the cold
application, but which lessened with returning
heat, and was promptly renewed by the repetition
of the remedy.

"The intolerable pain with which arthritic
inflammation is accompanied, was so perfectly
controllable in this case by reduced temperature,
that the patient kept it so constantly diminished
by its frequent use, as very speedily to subdue
it altogether. On the second day of its employ,
no disposition to return of pain on lengthening
the intervals of recurring to it continued. The
swelling and redness were also much decreased;
a livid hue indeed had superseded the florid aspect. The peculiar stiffness arising from debility,
and probably from more or less of serous effusion
in the cellular texture of the inflamed parts,
prevented either facility or strength of motion for
several days; but with the local disease terminated the systematic irritation, and every other
complaint.

"The patient waited on me at the distance of
several miles in the course of a week, to shew
the progress of his recovery, when bark, a nutri-
tious diet, friction, and bandage on the affected
limb, were farther directed. He soon after was
enabled

enabled to resume his active avocations without any inconvenience.

"This was a case of sheer gout, unmixed with any of those anomalies or irregularities which often obscure its evident character. The efficacy of the treatment rested on the anti-inflammant power of topical cold. The remedy was prompt, progressive, and unequivocal. The design of the medicine here employed was, by its diffusive exciting quality, to calm and harmonize the motive powers, to proportion duly the distribution of the circulating fluids, to balance the various secretions, and thereby to counteract either the formation or continuance of any sympathetically morbid action, which the pain of protracted gout is liable to occasion; but even this indication for the use of medicine is founded rather on extreme caution than on unquestionable necessity.

"Cases are in my recollection, in which the prejudices of theory would have shuddered to have hazarded a patient without a medicinal guard; but in which none was employed, and the event proved that none was requisite. One of this description is the following:

N "Case.

" Case 2 : A gentleman, who on the slightest catarrhal affection, from exposure to change of temperature, had been for many years subjected to podagral inflammation.—The great toe of one or both feet had been invariably the seat of the complaint. He was lately attacked on a journey, so as to be disabled from prosecuting it. Having learnt the good effect of my mode of treating gout, my advice was desired. The unprejudiced correctness of the patient's understanding induced him confidently to submit to the full force of reduced temperature. Cloths wetted in cold water were first applied in the evening, and renewed frequently throughout the ensuing night. The morbid heat yielded before the morning, and with that also the redness, tumefaction, and distempered sensibility. A sense of numbness, or rather weight only, was felt in the morning, which was no obstacle to the patient's pursuing his journey. Cold application was continued for a day or two, a ʳ ᵃ preventive. No farther complaint occurred, and the patient has not, to my knowledge, suffered from arthritic affection since that time. No medicine was directed. Every thing that tended to heat, by stimulating, was prohibited, and nothing more appeared to be necessary.

" This

" This is one among the numerous cases of rapid removal of arthritic inflammation by reduced temperature, which would perhaps almost constantly occur, were similar practice to be uniformly adopted. The earlier the mode of treatment is resorted to, the more speedily would the inflammatory affection be subdued, and consequently the danger (if any) of the irritation being transferred to any other part, be proportionately less, as sufficient time would not then be afforded for any associated or sympathetic movements to be generated, either generally or partially, in the system, which might possibly assume a similar action * on the cessation of the primary disease.

" The advantages also resulting from an early check being given to the disorder, consist in obviating change of structure in the vascular fabric of the affected parts, arising either from the generation of new vessels, the decomposition of the old, or from inorganic and obstructing effusions in the cellular texture.

* By "similar action" is to be understood inflammatory only : it could not be identically gouty, without having its seat in either the ligamentous or tendinous structure. K.

" Case

" Case 3. A gentleman, whose constitutional health had been long subjected to an habitual recurrence of podagral malady at uncertain intervals, and who had been lately benefited by the topical employ of diminished temperature under my direction, desired my advice in the earliest stage of an attack; so early indeed, as to be able to ride a distance of several miles to consult me. The great toe of one foot was then rapidly tumefying, highly heated, and becoming acutely painful; the foot and knee joints also partook of the irritation.

" The affected extremity was ordered to be enveloped in a cloth dipped in a cold fluid, consisting chiefly of water; but unimportantly disguised, both to obviate the probable alarm of the patient, and the certain *dread* of the family apothecary, who had distinguished himself as a very *Vulcan* by his *fiery ordinances* in the treatment of gout.

" The cold application allayed in a few hours the inflammatory symptoms, and its continuance speedily re-conducted the disordered action to the natural motive conditions of ease and health.

" This patient had never before a fit of the gout that did not confine him for several weeks; and

and if it be allowable to presume from the incipient violence of the last attack, its progressive
and permanent severity would have been at least
equal to what had been formerly experienced.
Its sudden repression and speedy removal, therefore, evince, in the most satisfactory manner,
that arthritic inflammation is indubitably a disease of excessive temperature; that its natural
antidote is diminished heat; that this remedy is
conveniently applied through the medium of
cold water; and that probably the most prompt
and efficacious mode of employing it would be
by either immersing the affected limb into that
fluid, or by incessant affusion with it *, until the
painful sense of morbid heat should wholly
subside.

"My experience fully warrants me in believ-
ing that this effect would almost invariably
happen in the course of a few hours.

* Since the publication of this remark, ample experience
has ascertained, that immersing the affected part is the most
expeditious, effectual, and commodious way of reducing gouty
inflammation, occurring on either the feet or hands. The
frequent renewal of cloths, dripping wet from the coldest water,
will answer every curative purpose on joints not conveniently
capable of being either immersed or affused. K.

N 3 "Case

"Case 4. A middle-aged man, by trade a mechanic, had been, during several years, periodically afflicted with gout. It usually attacked the feet, and occasionally also the hands. His accustomed confinement in this disorder, disabled him for a considerable length of time from engaging in his mechanical employment. At his last seizure (but a few weeks since) he desired my advice. The plan of treatment pursued in the preceding cases was commenced. The affected parts were assiduously plied with cold water, to which (as in every other instance) the pain speedily yielded; but if the renewal of cold was delayed beyond half an hour, distempered heat would return, accompanied, as the patient conceived, with an aggravated degree of irritation. The fluid, which was topically applied, was so slightly disguised, that it appeared too much like simple water not to awaken the patient's suspicion, and consequently his fear of its noxious repelling quality. This dread, by suitable explanation, however, was soon allayed, and a more unremitted continuance of cold application to the affected parts, completely subdued in a few days the several inflammations, leaving only the usual sense of debility and numbness, for which he was directed to use brisk friction, with a flesh-brush, two or three times

times a day. The camphorated tincture of opium (tinctura opii camphorata) and ammoniated tincture of guaiacum (tinctura guaiaci ammoniata) were also taken in doses of two drachms each, every four hours, in an aqueous vehicle, for the purpose of quieting the prevailing systematic irritation, and determining to the surface; an effect strongly indicated, to remedy an unvaried dryness of the skin.

" The patient called on me about a week after the cessation of his complaint, and discontinuance of all medicinal treatment, thanking me for the aid he had received, adding, that he had never before been freed from a fit of the gout so rapidly, with so little pain, and with so early a return of the natural powers of the affected parts.

" This case afforded me an opportunity of remarking, with much satisfaction, the perfect safety of reducing the inflammatory temperature of gouty affection, even in the worst state of constitutional health. A consumptive tendency was strikingly evident in the feebleness with which the ordinary functions of life were performed in this patient. Destitute of arterial tone and muscular vigour, and with that peculiarly dry and unyielding cough which characterizes

tubercular

tubercular irritation, the reactive powers of the system were extremely weak, and must have been overwhelmed, if, according to popular prejudice, the sudden allaying of arthritic inflammation could ever be followed by a morbid transference of it to some vital part of the system.

" This idea is really a mere *bugbear*, occasionally sanctioned even with the solemn gravity of medical erudition, which has served to alarm the prejudiced and the ignorant in every age, from remote antiquity, and to preclude the adoption of a rational mode of cure. The reverse of the prevailing opinion is true. It is not the early extinction of gouty inflammation that endangers a retrocession of morbid influence on the system, but its being protracted on a part.

" When, by long continuance, a local establishment of the disease is formed, it will ultimately diffuse its distempered action over the frame, and thus, by either generally or partially undermining, the motive powers of health become more or less predominant, according to circumstances of temperamental atony and susptibility for morbid impression.

" Case

" Case 5. This is an instance which may serve, *instar omnium*, as a decisive proof of perfect security in employing reduced temperature in external inflammation, whether purely arthritic, or as the *blending acumen* of the nosologist would denominate *rheumatismo-arthritic*, or any other description of inflammatory disorder. The subject of this case was a labouring man, who had repeatedly suffered from careless exposure to cold during the refrigerating influence of profuse perspiration. On a former occasion, severe peripneumony resulted from an abrupt reduction of temperature: in the instance under consideration, a violent inflammatory affection of every joint of both hands and feet was the consequence.

" The shining tumid aspect, and intolerable pain peculiar to the gout, induced a suspicion of its being that malady; but in the excessive temperature that prevailed, the distinction to me was no more than nominal.

" When inflammation is accompanied with a sense of heat literally *burning*, it is very unimportant what it is called; it is of more moment to repress its hurtful tendency with the utmost promptitude.

a

" This

" This patient's limbs were immediately enveloped with cloths dripping with cold water, which were renewed about every half hour. The moisture was detached by evaporation from the cloths as rapidly as if held before a fierce fire. The pain, as always happens, was speedily assuaged, but soon recurred, if not prevented by a timely renewal of cold; the constant application of which subdued by the following day the irritation of the feet and hands: when associated or sympathetic pain began to rage on the knees and shoulders, these parts soon became as inflamed and motionless as those which the irritation had relinquished. The same treatment was pursued, and with similar effect. The cessation of pain in these newly affected parts was the recommencement of it in those which were first diseased: thus did the irritation alternately change its position during several weeks. All this time the patient may be said to have been *soaked* in cold water.

" The pain was tolerable (scarcely indeed deserving the name) when the remedy was freely used; but either inattention, or fear of its proving mischievous, occasionally interrupted its due employ, to which probably the want of more early and decisive efficacy may be attributed. Latterly

Latterly it was judged right not only to reduce the heat of the parts actually inflamed, but also to keep those which had been recently relieved, in a state of diminished temperature. This expedient perfectly succeeded; no farther inflammation happened; and from that hour the alternate shifting of the inflammation ceased, and the patient began to recover his constitutional strength. No serious ailment occurred, at any stage of the disease, to the general health; nor did the occasional interposition of purgative, sudorific, and narcotic medicine in any degree mitigate the severity of the pain.

" Although a long series of recurring inflammation had broken and exhausted the constitutional strength, inducing that morbid state of irritability, which may be supposed to be peculiarly favourable to admitting diseased impressions, yet nothing like a transposition of the disordered excitement happened to any internal part of the system, and even under circumstances in which associative or sympathetic motions seemed to be performing the reciprocal office of *derivants* of irritation from the several affected parts. It would be difficult to adduce an example more strong than this, in testimony of the curative power of diminished heat in the worst
conditioned

conditioned instances of inflammation. It evinces, beyond all doubt, that excessive temperature is the *proximate cause*, and not merely a *symptom* or *effect*, of inflammation.

" How this is generated can only be known by investigating those distempered conditions of motive power, that occasion its morbid evolution and redundancy. This inquiry has long been with me a favourite speculation, and may probably hereafter, if leisure should permit, be sufficiently matured to warrant my submitting it to public consideration.

" I am, &c.

" Robert Kinglake."

" *Taunton,*
December 22, 1802.

An Address, by Dr. Kinglake.

" Dr. Kinglake presumes, from the *original view*, which he has submitted to the public, in his two papers on the *nature* and *cure* of *gout*, to request, *generally*, his medical brethren to communicate to him any intelligence, which correct experience might furnish, of the effects of his new mode of treatment, that he might be enabled, at no distant period, to present a mass of evidence

dence competent to determine, *beyond all doubt*, whether the arthritic patient must continue doomed to languish under the lingering and indefinite torture of an uncontrollable malady, or safely avail himself of a prompt and efficacious remedy.

" The conjoint aid of the medical faculty, in this investigation, is almost indispensably necessary, to countervail the insurmountable difficulties which would be opposed to a solitary endeavour, by the inveteracy of popular prejudice against the employ of *topical cold*, in an affection which has hitherto been supposed 'peculiarly to require an unremitted increase of both *local heat* and *systematic excitement*.

" *Taunton*,
December 22, 1802."

IV. *Mr. Wadd's Letter on the topical Use of cold Water in Gout.—Extracted from the Medical and Physical Journal, for the Year* 1803.

" To the Editors of the Medical and Physical Journal.

" Gentlemen,

" Not being a constant reader of your publication, I should not have seen Dr. Kinglake's

account

account of what he calls his 'new mode of 'treating the gout,' but for a medical friend, who shewed me the last number (No. 48) within these two days. I am greatly gratified that the subject is brought forward, and particularly so on account of the success the Doctor has had in persuading his arthritic patients to follow his advice.

" It is well known, in a large circle of my acquaintance, that I have made use of cold water, internally and externally, for the gout nearly twenty years* ; externally by wet cloths, and
immerging

---

* The testimony here given of gout having been familiarly checked by cold application, during nearly *twenty years*, refutes the opinion of the practice being fraught with injury to the health, at a more or less distant period. Popular prejudices always have, and always will exist; they are the unexamined adoptions of thoughtlessness; but it is more extraordinary for those who have been habituated to scientific inquiry, to attempt the justification of a received opinion, by every expedient which subtility can devise. This perverse artifice has been grossly exemplified with respect to the permanent preventive efficacy of vaccine inoculation against variolous infection. When its immediate preventive power became incontestable, the acuteness, or rather *virulence* of prejudice, foresaw that the effect could not be lasting; and under the secure shelter of *inscrutable futurity*, it was as presumptuously as ignorantly asserted, that the vaccinated constitution would be again susceptible of variolous infection in the course of *three years :* this time elapsed, the prediction was
falsified.

Immerging the limb in the approach, and every stage of the fit. I have even exhibited before medical men of the first eminence, and gentlemen of sense not of the profession, but subject to the disease. By the first I have been pronounced *rash*, and by the last called *bold*; but unfortunately cannot boast of a single convert. Whenever opportunity offered I have argued the rationality of the practice, it being a favourite topic, and maintained it on the theory I had imbibed of the disease, and which I have been strongly urged to put into print, but have been

falsified. The time was then said to have been too short, and that *five years* were necessary to wear out the vaccine influence. A similar scheme of reasoning and prophecy has been resorted to relative to the refrigerant treatment of gout. At first, a *very war-whoop* was raised against it; oh! it would infallibly destroy in a *few hours*. The treatment was applied, no destruction ensued, the patient became instantly relieved, soon cured, and afterwards enjoyed a much better state of general health than was usually experienced after the spontaneous departure of the disease. This is *strange!* but, however, it does not invalidate the *principle*, exclaims the *pseudo-prophet;* that is still *just*; the error was in time only; the destructive influence, it is seen, cannot be quite so *rapid*; but without fear of disappointment, it *will*, it *must* occur (or the prejudice is *good for nothing*) at some indefinite period, from *six months* to *two years*, beyond which time the annals of *repelled gout* are challenged to adduce a single instance of any one having survived, if he had been subjected to the deadly treatment. What, not a *single survivor* on record? why, there are already *hundreds* who might be brought forward, if necessary, in utter refutation of this ignorant, malevolent, and *secundum artem* killing prejudice.　K.

deterred, lest the words rash and bold should be changed into *mad*.

"Thank God, I have not paid the debt so long predicted by my brethren of the faculty; and I pray for long life; for, should my death happen short of ninety, it will be attributed to the use of cold water in the gout, and may prevent me Christian burial, so strong is prejudice.

"I beg, Gentlemen, you will accept of an apology for not being more acquainted with your useful work. I have not yet seen the beginning of this subject in No. 33, but I shall not lose sight of that, and what may appear hereafter. I was willing to be thus early in the field to countenance the good work, and may come forth again when I can corroborate my opinion by that of others. I am now creeping out of the severest fit I ever had; I plunged the limb into cold water at the height of the inflammation, when pain was excessive, and not to be subdued by opium. I obtained temporary ease *.

"*Basinghall Street, London,*   I am, &c.
   Feb. 14, 1803.   "S. WADD."

* This temporary ease might have been extended to a permanent cure, if the affected limb had been kept sufficiently long under cold water to have fully reduced the inflammatory heat. A mere *plunge* is widely inadequate to that effect.   K.

V. *An*

V. *An anonymous Attack, signed " Constant Reader," on Dr. Kinglake's Mode of treating Gout.—Extracted from the Medical and Physical Journal for the Year 1803.*

" To the Editors of the Medical and Physical Journal.

" Gentlemen,

" Permit to say, that Dr. Kinglake's use of cold water in the gout is not so new, and peculiar to himself, as he appears to imagine. The illustrious Harvey, discoverer of the circulation, used to plunge his feet into cold water to mitigate the severity of painful paroxysms of that disease. It has even been said, that he shortened his life by that practice *.

" As Dr. K. calls loudly upon his medical brethren to communicate any observations which may enable him to make up his mind as soon as possible, the following case, on the authenticity of which he may depend, is much at his service.

---

* Who says so? This *gout-killing incognito writer.* It will be hereafter proved, whoever he may be, that he has forfeited all claim to *credit*, by an egregious misrepresentation, which has every appearance of being *intentional.*   K.

" The

" The late celebrated Dr. Gregory, of Edinburgh, father of the present Professor of Medicine
in that university, was very liable to gout. A
friend of the present writer called on him one
evening, and found him bathing his feet in cold
water *. He observed to the Doctor, that he was
doing what he would hardly recommend to his
patients. ‘ No,’ said the Doctor; ‘ but this appli-
‘ cation mitigates pain, which I am unwilling to
‘ bear, and I have hitherto experienced no bad
‘ effects from it.’ The next morning, the Doctor,
to the regret of every admirer of science, and of
professional liberality, was found lifeless in his
bed.

" But why trouble ourselves any farther about
the gout ? One gentleman can completely pump
out the gout from the system in a day or two,
and another has discovered a remedy, a few
spoonsful of which will enable a cripple to rise
from his bed, put on a pair of tight shoes, eat a
good dinner, and afterwards dance a hornpipe.
Surely one remedy for a disease is sufficient; my
only fear is, that, unless we can find out some

* It will be seen hereafter, by Drs. Duncan's refutation, that
instead of *cold water* having ever been used, much solicitude was
shewn to keep the feet *warm*; which evinces this case to be
altogether a most *vile fabrication.* K.

new

new diseases, for which as yet there are no remedies, the faculty must starve!

" A Constant Reader."

VI. *Dr. Kinglake's Reply to " Constant Reader,"
and to Mr. Wadd.—Extracted from the Medical
and Physical Journal for the Year 1809.*

" To the Editors of the Medical and Physical
Journal.

" Gentlemen,

" Not a page of your useful Journal should be
misemployed, in giving place to any animadver-
sions from me, on the attack which your
" Constant Reader" has made, in your last number, on my mode of treating gout, did it not
derive some claim to notice, both from your
having admitted it into your publication, and
from the discouraging impression it may possibly
make on the timid and the prejudiced.

" It must be readily perceived, that the communication breathes a spirit of levity and wrangling, wholly inconsistent with the grave decorum
due to the investigation and decision of a philosophical subject; nor does the veil of anonymous

O 2   concealment,

concealment, which the author has thought fit to assume, impart to the statement the genuine stamp of unquestionable authenticity.

" *Hearsay reports* are not legitimate documents for determining the merits of scientific inquiry. What principle, in either physics or morals, would be secure, if assailable by the detracting insinuations of adverse and unsubstantiated rumour?

" The names of Harvey and Gregory are adduced to discredit a practice which their superior intelligence led them to adopt in their own cases. Could a stronger proof be given of the firm persuasion they had of its salutary powers? Nor is the supposed shade of the narrative its gloomy part, for it is not pretended that either of these eminent men ever repented what they had done, or in any degree disparaged its beneficial efficacy.

" If trembling spectators and commentators, like your ' Constant Reader,' should imagine dangers where none exist, and assign causes for deaths which not even a *casual coincidence* of circumstances fully warrants, such groundless dread ought not to repress a humane endeavour to in-

culcate

culcate a rational mode of curing an hitherto untractable malady.

" It has never been my object to assume credit for either originality or peculiarity, in reducing the morbid excess of temperature in arthritic affection by diminished heat. It is impossible the principle should have escaped the earliest reasoning on the subject. The principle of the practice may therefore be rather considered as *common* to human intelligence than *peculiar* to any individual.

" The doctrine of distempered heat at once pervades and constitutes the most intelligent and instructive parts of Hippocrates's writings. The medical principles and practice of Sydenham also, founded on temperature, formed a transcendent epoch in the history of curative medicine; and, happily for mankind, finally overthrew the fatal delusions of humoral pathology and alexipharmic jargon.

" Conducted then by analogy, it occurred to me as highly reasonable that gout, distinguished like other inflammations by excessive heat, and marked by no essential difference, might be subdued in a similar manner. This persuasion in-

o 3

duced

duced me to assimilate the treatment. Not a single fact had previously reached my knowledge to authorize the trial; though undoubtedly many were extant. To me, therefore, the practice was relatively, though not absolutely, original. The only claim to originality, which seems to exist in my right, and the only one which deserves a moment's solicitude to establish, is that of publicly recommending the practice, after having experienced its salutary effects in numerous instances, in which the treatment was conducted with such disguise and secrecy as were necessary to obviate the prohibitive influence of prevailing prejudices against it.

" In my estimation, nothing can be more degradingly futile, or ridiculously absurd, than capriciously cavilling at a fair attempt to be useful, or to deny merit to those who, at all risks, aim at a practical improvement by patient experiment, and respectful publication of the result.

" Your correspondent, Mr. Wadd, has my implicit credit in averring his long familiarity with the topical use of cold water in the cure of gout; but how is his zeal for the improvement of the healing art to be appreciated, if, confident of the salutary powers of reduced temperature in

4

that disorder, he did not boldly adopt it in his private practice, and recommend it to public attention?

" He says he could never prevail on any patient to submit to the treatment. It was not likely that he should. What patient will accede to a proposed remedy, that has the reputation of being *certainly* pernicious?

" The efficacy of the treatment might have been subjected to the test of experiment, without alarming existing prejudices. Indeed, it should be an invariable rule, in investigating the effects of a new remedy, cautiously to conceal the nature and object of the trial, to prevent its specific operation being disguised by the influence of imagination.

" Since my last communication on the cure of arthritis, the previous stock of my experience has received considerable addition from correspondents, bearing the strongest testimony to the speedy, safe, and effectual remedy afforded to gout, by the application of cold water. One case has also since occurred, in my own practice, more violently, extensively, and critically circumstanced than any former instance in my

observation,

observation, in which the incessant employ of cold water, partly by bathing and partly by keeping the affected joints enveloped with cloths wetted in that fluid, completely extinguished the arthritic temperature, and restored the inflamed parts to perfect ease, and tolerable motion, in the course of three days. Friction has since fully renovated the motive power.

" Firmly convinced of the inestimable benefit that will accrue to mankind from a *liberal* investigation of the curative power of topical cold in arthritic inflammation, the medical faculty will excuse my again soliciting the earliest intelligence of their experience on the subject, that an opportunity may soon be afforded me of presenting the public with such information, as will unequivocally prove gout, like all other descriptions of inflammation, to be a disease of *excessive temperature*, and, agreeably to an evident law of nature, most appropriately, promptly, and efficaciously remediable by *diminished heat*. Time will elucidate and confirm this opinion.

'Magna est veritas, et prævalebit.'

" I am, &c.

" ROBERT KINGLAKE."

" *Taunton*,
April 9, 1803.

VII.

VII. *Extract of a Letter from Dr. Hall to Dr. Kinglake, relative to the Mistatement in the above-cited anonymous Attack, signed " Constant Reader," on Dr. Kinglake's Mode of treating Gout.*

" To Dr. Kinglake, Taunton.

" Dear Sir,

" It gives me great satisfaction to learn, that a practice, which I am fully persuaded must ultimately prove of the most extensive benefit to arthritic patients, seems likely, at no very distant period, to be established on the solid basis of experience and observation : an event which, reasoning from the dislike to innovation, unfortunately but too prevalent, even among some of the more enlightened members of the profession, I was scarcely sanguine enough to expect.

" I am glad to observe that Drs. Duncan have, in their last year's Annals, positively contradicted the assertion made in the Medical and Physical Journal, respecting the manner of the late Dr. Gregory's death. Not that any such coincidence would have, in my mind, operated against the employment of topical refrigeration; but because I am fully aware how much mischief is frequently

quently done to the cause of science, by incautious assertions, or arguments addressed to the passions and prejudices of mankind. Nothing has, in my opinion, proved more injurious to the practice of medicine than connecting as cause and effect, circumstances which have no relation to each other, merely because they happen to fall out together, or are merely simultaneous. *Post hoc, ergo propter hoc*, is certainly a very unphilosophical mode of argumentation, and cannot be relied on, though it has not unfrequently led to the rejection of a practice, which a more enlarged experience has afterwards demonstrated to be useful.

" Permit me, dear Sir, to reiterate my best wishes for the success of your benevolent labours, and to assure you,

" I am,

" With the greatest respect, &c.

" R. HALL, M. D."

" *Church Row, Hampstead,*
July 24, 1803.

VIII.

VIII. *Extract of the Passage alluded to by Dr. Hall, from Drs. Duncan's Annals of Medicine for the last Year.—Published by Dr. Kinglake in the Medical and Physical Journal for the Year 1803, as a " Correction of a Mistatement."*

" To the Editors of the Medical and Physical Journal.

" Gentlemen,

" In the true spirit of just investigation, you have, as liberally as laudably, endeavoured to discourage the communications of anonymous writers, by refusing them the authority of medical evidence. You will therefore readily coincide with me in the propriety of correcting the misrepresentation contained in a paper of your Journal (No. 50, p. 360), signed ' Constant Reader,' by publishing the subsequent remarks on that subject, extracted from the last volume of Drs. Duncan's Annals of Medicine. Indeed it would be compromising a gross mistatement to withhold this intelligence from your numerous readers. The paper alluded to, appeared to me, *prima facie*, to be as exceptionable for its want of internal as external evidence. My own words, in reply to the author, bear testimony to this opinion. These were, ' It must be readily per-
' ceived, that the communication (in question)
' breathes

' breathes a spirit of levity and wrangling wholly
' inconsistent with the grave decorum due to the
' investigation and decision of a philosophical
' subject; nor does the veil of anonymous con-
' cealment, which the author has thought fit
' to assume, impart to the statement the genuine
' stamp of unquestionable authenticity.'

"It will be clearly seen how commendably
the scientific labours of the authors of the Annals
of Medicine are regulated by a scrupulous attention to the interests of truth and philosophical
impartiality, by the following extract, in which
they discover a solicitude to rectify a mistake,
which, if unexplained, may have operated to the
prejudice of a doctrine they profess rather to dis-
approve than to defend.

*Extract of an Article in the last Volume of Drs.
Duncan's Annals of Medicine, entitled, "Notice
of Dr. Kinglake's Proposal of the topical Use of
cold Water in the Gout."*

The following Letter, addressed to the Editors
of the Medical and Physical Journal, has appeared in the 50th Number of that Publication.

"Gentlemen,

"As Dr. Kinglake calls loudly on his medical brethren to communicate any observations
which

which may enable him to make up his mind as soon as possible, the following case, on the authenticity of which he may depend, is much at his service.

" The late celebrated Dr. Gregory, of Edin-burgh, father of the present Professor of Medicine in that university, was very liable to gout. A friend of the present writer called on him one evening, and found him bathing his feet in cold water. He observed to the Doctor, that he was doing what he would hardly recommend to his patients. ' No,' said the Doctor; ' but this appli-' cation mitigates pain, which I am unwilling to ' bear, and I have hitherto experienced no bad ' effects from it.' The next morning the Doctor, to the regret of every admirer of science and of pro-fessional liberality, was found lifeless in his bed.

" But why trouble ourselves any farther about the gout ? One gentleman can completely pump out the gout from the system in a day or two; and another has discovered a remedy, a few spoonsful of which will enable the cripple to rise from his bed, put on a pair of tight shoes, eat a good dinner, and afterwards dance an hornpipe. Surely one remedy for a disease is sufficient; my only fear is, that, unless we can find out some

new

new diseases, for which as yet there are no remedies, the faculty must starve!

       " A Constant Reader."

 " Although, from the conclusion of this letter,
it is evident that the writer of it means to treat
Dr. Kinglake's proposal with ridicule, yet it will
naturally be concluded, that what he has asserted
respecting the late Dr. Gregory is strictly true;
and, if true, it would certainly have been an
important fact. It was indeed a very current report at the time of Dr. Gregory's death, that he
had been accustomed to bathe his feet in cold
water, and had done so the evening before that
event took place. But upon the authority of
those who had the best opportunities of knowing, we can inform the public that this report is
entirely groundless; that, on the contrary, Dr.
Gregory, who had often been subjected to severe
attacks of the gout, was at much pains to keep
his feet warm *; that he had no symptoms of

               gout

---

 * " At much pains to keep his feet warm!" How does
Constant Reader reconcile this *important fact* with his grave
assertion, that a friend of his had *actually* " found the Doctor
bathing his feet in cold water," and been *eye-witness* to the
transaction! It cannot be, *such* falsehood does not exist. This
alleged, or rather *feigned* friend, merely *echoed* the vulgar report;
Constant Reader *adeptly* added the remainder. Thus truth, sacred
               truth,

gout for many months before his death, having
enjoyed a much longer interval of health than
usual ; that on the very day preceding his death
he had dined abroad with some friends, and had
supped with his family ; that he had not bathed
his feet the night before he died; and was left by
his son, the present Dr. Gregory, at half an hour
after twelve o'clock, preparing his lecture for
the next day, and apparently in perfect health ;
but was found lifeless next morning ; and that,
from the undisturbed condition of the bed-
clothes, it was concluded he had died without a
struggle."

The Editors then proceed to say, " But although the sudden death of Dr. Gregory affords
no objection against Dr. Kinglake's proposal,
yet we are very far from asserting that the application of cold wet cloths to a part inflamed and
painful from gout, is a safe practice *."

truth, has to combat the manifold disguises and artifices of malevolent misrepresentation. May its interests never be less vic-
torious than on the present occasion ! K.

* This opinion results from prejudice, but may justly boast
the support of *dignified* and *inflexible integrity*. It never will, nor
ever should be surrendered, but on the clearest conviction of its
being groundless. It will then be abandoned with an *honest
candour*, that will exhibit an *amiable contrast* to the *malignant
calumny* of Constant Reader. K.

" Such

" Such is the refutation which a zealous and unbiassed love of scientific truth has enabled me to quote on 'Constant Reader's' unqualified assertion, that his statement of Dr. Gregory's case possessed an *"authenticity on which he* (Dr. Kinglake) *may depend." 'Humanum est errare.'*

"I am, &c.

"*Taunton,*   "ROBERT KINGLAKE."
October 23, 1803.

———

Messrs. Scott and Taynton on cold Applications in Gout.—Published in the Medical and Physical Journal for the Year 1803.

" To the Editors of the Medical and Physical Journal.

"Gentlemen,

"In consequence of Dr. Kinglake's pressing invitation to medical men, to communicate their experience in the use of cold applications in the cure of gout and rheumatism, Mr. *Scott* and Mr. *Taynton*, surgeons, at *Bromley*, in *Kent*, cannot any longer defer making known through the medium of your excellent publication, the result of their own practice in these disorders.

Amongst

Amongst several cases that have fallen under their care, they think the four following the most deserving of notice.

CASE I.

" On the 24th of February 1803, they were sent for to a young married woman, who had been ill three days. She was unable to stir hand or foot; her pulse was quick and hard; she had great thirst, and complained of severe pain in her feet and ankles, attended with swelling and inflammation; the wrists and elbows were also affected. Cloths wetted in a solution of muriated ammonia were ordered to be constantly applied to the parts, and one grain of opium was given her at night. On the 29th they were agreeably surprised to find the swelling and inflammation nearly gone, and the pains much abated. On the 26th she was able to walk down stairs, and by the beginning of March was cured.

CASE II.

" On the 14th of April they visited a young man, labouring under acute rheumatism. The febrile symptoms were pretty severe; he was unable to walk, felt great pain in the ankles and knees, and in one elbow. As he was costive, he was ordered to take an opening medicine, and to apply constantly the cold solution. He soon experienced ease; and though the pains shifted from one joint to another, and the weakness did not leave him so soon as in the former case, he was able to move about with the assistance of crutches in three days, and by the 28th was well.

CASE III.

" A gentleman's butler was attacked with gout in the great toe of his left foot, on the 11th of April in the morning. He had repeated exacerbations and remissions of pain till the 14th when they saw him: they found the toe greatly inflamed, the skin shining, the parts exquisitely tender, and the patient not able to set his foot to the ground. It was wrapped up in flannel, which was immediately removed, and in its stead it was surrounded with wet cloths dipped in the cold solution, and an opening draught was given him. He found relief in half an hour, and on the following day could put his foot to the ground. On the 20th he was quite well.

CASE IV.

" A lady upwards of sixty, habitually subject to the asthma, and tedious fits of the gout,

whilst

whilst labouring under severe dyspnœa and cough, attended with pyrexia, was attacked with pain and inflammation in the instep and joint of the great toe. The parts were of course immediately enveloped by her attendants in a quantity of flannel, with a view, *no doubt*, of enticing all her other *complaints on this one spot.* The cough was treated as if she had no gout, and the gout as if she had had no cough. The cold application was of great use; no unpleasant symptom occurred, and she was soon cured.

" *Mr. Scott* and *Mr. Taynton* take this opportunity of returning their acknowledgment to *Dr. Kinglake* for his valuable communication on this subject. They have every reason to think that his plan of treatment will prove highly beneficial to mankind; and as they are in very extensive practice, they will neglect no opportunity of giving it a fair trial, and of making known the result of their failure, as well as of their success *.

" *Bromley, Kent,*
May 12, 1803."

Extract

---

* To such liberal investigators of practical medicine, the best interests of the healing art may be safely confided. The cause of the refrigerant treatment of gout will no doubt derive

much

Extract of a Letter on cold Bathing in Rheumatism, published in the Medical and Physical Journal for the Year 1803. Signed *S. G.*

" To the Editors of the Medical and Physical Journal.

" Gentlemen,

" The case I have to offer you is sterling, it is of my own person.

" Nearly two years ago, after a day of great fatigue, I had occasion to walk, *au soir*, over a considerable extent of pasturage land, the grass of which was wet. I had not proceeded far, before I began to feel uneasiness in my right ankle and foot, which, before the end of my ambulation, became so very painful, that I was unable to walk without frequent haltings.

much additional support from their useful and exemplary labours. Indeed it is to be regretted that their laudable scheme of inquiry has not been more generally imitated. In that case, gout would by this time have been stripped of its *ideal terrors*, would have nakedly appeared in its true character of *simple inflammation*, and would have been as promptly and safely cured by the topical application of cold. This *important fact*, however slowly, will ultimately be established.

" I ob-

"I obtained no remedy from rest, for the next day the complaint appeared to be aggravated. The foot was swollen and turned awry, bending inwardly; this deformity was so great, that a medical acquaintance affirmed there must be a luxation of the bone. I knew however the complaint was only muscular. The ankle and foot were coloured with a rheumatic redness. In a few weeks erratic rheumatism afflicted every joint of my body. I had sometimes lumbago, at other times rheumatism in my shoulders, so badly, that it was with difficulty I could put on my coat; in my wrist, that I could not supinate my hand; in my knuckles, that I could not pare an apple. In truth, for upwards of a year, I was lame and decrepit. To be plain, my infirmities began at last to acquire me the odious appellation of 'The Lame Doctor.' You may justly suppose I was very solicitous to get rid of my vexatious companion, rheumatism.

"I used most of the medicines commonly prescribed for that disease, and also electricity. As for electricity, I should have been equally benefited had I merely rotated the electrical wheel. It is worth remarking, that soon after the accession of rheumatism I removed to another part of

the

the globe, I dwelled four months within the tropic of Cancer; yet a hot climate, and all the medicines I had taken, did not procure me a remission of the disease. Returning to England in May last, I determined to try the effect of immersions into cold spring water. I continued indefatigably the use of the immersions for nearly four months; I constanly bathed once, frequently twice, and sometimes three times a day. At each immersion I usually swam about in the water for a few minutes. For the first month the bathing seemed to have no other effect on me than a remission of rheumatism while I was in the water. In the course of the second month I was much encouraged to proceed in my cold plan. At last I relinquished the bathing, because it was unnecessary to seek farther, for what I had already found, a *perfect recovery.*

" It may be proper to observe that during the bathing I adopted the use of fleecy hosiery stockings, which I believe materially assisted in the completion of the cure. I shall be cautious of betraying the sciolist, shall assume no principle, nor involve confidence with this case, which in my experience is a solitary fact. This case was

such

such as I have here related. If you think it will add to the stock of useful information, you are welcome to print this letter *.

" I am, &c.

" S. G."

" *April 8th,* 1802.

On the beneficial Effects of reduced Temperature in gouty Complaints, by R. O. Millett, Jun.— Extracted from the Medical and Physical Journal for the Year 1803.

" To the Editors of the Medical and Physical Journal.

" Gentlemen,

" Several instances of the beneficial effects of reduced temperature for the removal of gouty

---

* Although no anonymous communication is entitled to *unquestionable credit,* yet the strong internal evidence of truth afforded in this statement, may be admitted in support of the doctrine advanced in the preceding dissertation; namely, that every degree of morbid excitement of the ligamentous and tendinous structure, whether going the length of positive inflammation, or assuming only the more transient form of shifting irritation, is *proximately* caused by excessive temperature; that it must therefore be necessarily aggravated by increased heat, whether from climate, regimen, or topical application; and that its appropriate, direct, and effectual cure (if curable), is only sooner or later attainable by refrigerant treatment.   K.

complaints,

complaints; which have appeared in the Medical and Physical Journal, and Dr. Kinglake's request to medical men, to make known their intelligence on the subject, have induced me to communicate the following case.

" Moses Simons, aged fifty-four, accustomed to a very liberal use of spirituous liquors, had been afflicted with gout generally three or four times a year, for ten years, sometimes in his hands, and other times in his knees, but his ankles and toes chiefly suffered; when those parts were attacked, they swelled, inflamed, and had a glossy appearance, attended with a burning sensation; sometimes his head and stomach were also affected with pains, and the latter with nausea and dyspepsia.

" About two years ago, when his toes happened to be affected with gout, a neighbour of his (not a medical man) called to see him, and advised him to hold his foot under a cock of cold water; by the help of a stick, he with difficulty walked about a hundred yards, and kept his foot for ten minutes under a large cock, from which, cold water was poured with great force; during which time, he heard a crackling

4

nbise * issuing from his foot, and found such immediate relief, that he threw aside his stick, and walked to his house with ease, and has not since had any return of gout, or symptoms of it, unless an extensive ·livid-coloured inflammation, with very little tumour, which took place a year ago in his left hypochondriac region, may be considered of that nature. As this inflammation remained stationary for several days, he sent for me; I thought it might not suppurate, and after he had taken some laxatives, it subsided without desquamation of the cuticle; a fortnight afterwards, another inflammation took place in his arm, which soon became hard and pointed, as a phlegmon; warm poultices were applied, and it suppurated, forming several deep holes, which, as soon as he could be prevailed upon, I laid open into one wound, and it healed in two months time; the use of his arm is quite restored, and he is very well in every respect, and continues in his employment in the copperworks, where he has been for ten years exposed

---

* Was not this sound occasioned by the vibratory percussion of repulsive motion or heat in its rapid evolution and escape from the inflamed part, through the comparatively low temperature of cold water? and is it not similar to the hissing effect produced by the contact of that fluid with an ignited substance? K.

to

to great heat, and the sudden application of cold when in perspirption, and inhaling the most noisome effluvia proceeding from the furnace *.

"I am, &c.

"R. O. Millett, Jun."

"*Hayle, Cornwall,*
July 28th, 1803.

* Though the latter part of this case is not materially relevant to the former, yet it has been thought proper to state it at length, lest it should be surmised, that it had been disingenuously withheld, as tending to involve the credit of the cooling treatment. The very reverse appears to me to be the fact. It proves in a manner almost singular, the immediate and permanent efficacy of diminished heat in gouty affection. The subsequent inflammations seemed to have been purely accidental, at least to have had no *intelligible* connexion with cured gout. They were mild determinations to the cuticular surface, neither marked with any virulent symptom, nor accompanied with any sympathetic affection of the ligaments and tendons, *the exclusive seat of gouty inflammation.* The durable cessation of gout in this case, evinces a complete annihilation of that *distempered excitability* of the ligamentous and tendinous structure, which the protracted disease so constantly entails, and but too often irrecoverably establishes. This entire freedom from painful disease justly improves the *prospect* of future health, and renders the *dread* of consequent disorder as futile as it is impossible. K.

On

On the good Effects of diminished Temperature in a Case of Rheumatism, signed E. O.—Extracted from the Medical and Physical Journal for the Year 1803.

" To the Editors of the Medical and Physical Journal.

" Gentlemen,

" Through the medium of your excellent publication, I learnt the successful result of the practice of Dr. Kinglake, in arthritic complaints, by diminshed temperature ; I have therefore taken the liberty of submitting the following case of rheumatism for your consideration, treated in a similar manner.

" T. G. a seaman of one of his Majesty's ships, aged twenty-three, while cruising on the coast of France, in very hazy weather, was attacked in the evening of the second of last June, with general acute pains in the limbs and head ; great heat and thirst, pulse quick and full. I immediately took sixteen ounces of blood from the arm, and administered the following bolus :

R Pulv. antim. (P. L.) gra. iii.
Calomel. gra. v.
Confect. damoc. q. s. fiat bolus, hora somni sumendus.

3d,

" 3d. A profuse perspiration in the course of the night relieved, in a tolerable degree, the pains in the upper extremities, but those of the lower ones were augmented, together with one ankle and knee swollen, and considerably inflamed. Head easy, thirst and general indisposition continued, proceeding, I imagined, from the excruciating pain which existed in the lower extremities.

" I enveloped them with cloths wet with cold salt water, which from the excessive temperature reigning, I was obliged to get renewed about every fifteen minutes, as the moisture evaporated as quickly as if they had been exposed to a fire. Administered Pulv. ipecac. comp. hora somni.

" 4th. Upper extremities perfectly easy, the lower ones considerably relieved; inflammation of knee and ankle very much diminished; skin moist, pulse soft, bowels regular, &c. Continued the cold as before, and repeated the Pulv. ipecac. comp. at bed-time,

" 5th. Rested well during the night; phlegmon removed, and tumefaction nearly so. Pain in lower extremities was very trifling; pulse
- regular,

regular, appetite good. I persevered in the use of the same remedies.

" 6th. Lower extremities perfectly free from pain. Repet. remedia.

" 7th. In the morning was free from complaint, excepting debility; but in the course of the day his wrists became painful, tumefied, and inflamed. I immediately enveloped *them* in the same manner I had done the knees and ankles. Rep. Pulv. ipecac. comp. ut antea.

" 8th. Pains in the wrists relieved, and the inflammation and swelling disappeared. Persevered in the use of cold water and powder. It is necessary to observe that I continued the cold applications to the knees and ankles, in order to prevent a sympathetic return *.

" 9th. Free from complaints, except debility, and a stiffness of lower limbs, which I ordered

---

* This precaution was highly judicious. It will in general be found effectually to avail, in obviating both original and sympathetic relapses, by salutarily repressing the strong tendency to a renewal of excessive temperature in the parts, which have been recently agitated and distempered by inflammatory excitement. K.

to

to be rubbed gently with a flesh-brush, and gave him half a drachm of powdered bark mixed with wine, four times a day. From this time he began to recover his health and strength, and on the 16th returned to his duty.

" I beg leave to observe, that this man, about two years ago, was attacked in a similar way, and was confined to his bed for six weeks, unable to raise either *hand* or *foot*; and I have every reason to believe, from the violence of the attack, that I should have had him confined for the same length of time, if not longer, had I pursued the usual method of cure practised on these occasions; but the sensible and judicious *practice* of Dr. Kinglake in arthritic complaints, pointed out to me a remedy at once effectual, speedy, and *cheap*, for the relief of one of the most painful and tedious complaints incident to the human body, and a complaint that is extremely prevalent in his Majesty's navy, particularly when employed in the Channel service.

" Before I had an opportunity, owing to an unavoidable absence from my native country, of reading any of your well-conducted Journals, I had been in the habit of making use of cold water in local affections of the joints with con-
                                    siderable

siderable advantage; I therefore with a tolerable confidence hesitated not applying it in the above case.

"If you think this single testimony will tend in the smallest degree to corroborate the evidence of your able correspondent in the safety and propriety of using diminished temperature for the relief of painful and inflammatory affections of the joints, whether called by the name of rheumatism or gout, you are perfectly at liberty to make what use of it you may deem fit; and if *perchance* it should merit your notice, it will amply satisfy your attentive reader *

"E. O."

---

* This case affords a very interesting detail of that description of ligamentous and tendinous inflammation, usually termed *rheumatism*, in contradistinction to that which is denominated gout. It has been held in the preceding view of the subject, that the difference is only nominal, that they are but different appellations for an inflammatory excitement of the same structure. Every variety indeed may occur in the degree of violence with which the disease may prevail; but this creates no *radical* change in its *identical* nature. Hence the treatment is correctly assimilated; and it will be found to produce the same beneficial effects, however variously the affection may be named. The superior value of this communication induced me to procure it; the *authenticity* of a real signature, which was given as follows, with a liberality worthy of *truth*, and a laudable zeal for medical improvement. K.

Dr.

Dr. Kinglake's Request for the real Signature of E. O.—Extracted from the Medical and Physical Journal for the Year 1803.

" To the Editors of the Medical and Physical Journal.

" Gentlemen,

" The communication in your last number, subscribed E. O. on the salutary effects of reduced temperature in rheumatic or gouty affection, is so pointedly in support of the treatment proposed by me, for the prompt and effectual cure of that malady, as to induce me to trouble you to request of the author his real signature, that no possible suspicion may attach to its authenticity, from its appearing anonymously. Such a detail of facts is truly valuable, and should possess every external claim to implicit admission as correct medical evidence.

" A knowledge of the intelligent author's name will enable me to incorporate his case with many others in an appendix to a work on gout, now preparing by me for speedy publication. In the mean time the transmission either to your Journal or to myself, of any farther experience on this interesting subject, cannot fail to extend and improve the object of my inquiry.

" The

" The success of the treatment under my own direction continues to exceed my most sanguine expectation, and promises soon to acquire it a very general and confident adoption.

" I am, &c.

" *Taunton,*　　　　　　" ROBERT KINGLAKE."
September 8th, 1803.

E. O.'s real Signature communicated to Dr. King-lake, in the following Letter.

" Sir,

"On looking over the Medical Journal for the month of October, which only reached me a few days ago, in consequence of my being absent on a cruise in the Channel for these last four months, I observed a letter from you, announcing the very flattering attention you paid to a case with diffidence communicated to the Editors of that work, upon the good effects of diminished temperature in rheumatism. I am well aware, Sir, that *initials* are tantamount to *anonymous,* consequently cannot be admitted as complete medical evidence; but being a young surgeon, and not in the habit of submitting any remarks to the criticising world, I felt a backwardness in giving my real signature, yet was desirous to make the case public, in order to assist in recommending a mode of cure in a very painful complaint, which *à priori* might appear to preju-

Q

diced

diced minds as repugnant to reason; therefore, in order to remove all kind of suspicion as to the authenticity of the case recorded, I with cheerfulness subscribe my *full signature* for any use you may think proper to apply it; and beg leave to assure you that from the success you have already had, it is my intention to pursue the practice with as much perseverance and attention as my situation at present will admit of, being confident in my own mind of its propriety, and shall feel a pleasure in having the honour of repeating to you my proceedings.

"Since the case already recorded, nothing has offered. Within these three days I have been trying the effects of cold water in a case of lumbago, from which, as yet, no benefit has arisen, and I fear I shall be obliged to desist from its use; for whenever the application is renewed, a general shivering takes place. However, I shall continue the plan for twenty-four hours longer, being desirous of giving it a fair trial *.

  "I remain, Sir,
   "With every wish for your welfare,
"*His Majesty's Ship* "Yours with respect,
  Alcmene,   "EDWARD OWEN."
"*Guernsey, Nov.* 24*th,* 1803.

* Unless there should be a considerable degree of local tumefaction and heat, in a case of *lumbago, general* cold bathing
               promises

Observations on the beneficial Effects of reduced Temperature in gouty and rheumatic Inflammation, by J. Ricards.—Extracted from the Medical and Physical Journal for the Year 1803.

" A few months since, some observations were made by the reporter, respecting applications of a cold nature to local inflammations of a specific kind, as gout and rheumatism, which are generally considered as diseases whose existence should be rather encouraged than repelled, and which are thus very commonly protracted to a very tedious length.

" We are much indebted to a physician of great discrimination and ability (Dr. Kinglake), for the remarks and relation of facts on this subject, which have been recently presented to the public by the medium of the Medical and Physical Journal, and whose assiduity in the collection of well-substantiated cases, in which

promises to prove more salutary than the topical application of cold water; but if the lumbar vertebral ligaments should be highly inflamed, attended with external swelling, redness, and exquisite sensibility on pressure, the case is then *sheer gout*, and should be combated with unremitting refrigeration, until the inflammatory temperature be totally subdued.   K.

similar

similar treatment has been pursued with success, will in all probability add much to our knowledge with respect to the nature of these diseases, and to our capability in the removal or mitigation of them.

" Several cases have come within my knowledge, since those which have been already alluded to, in which the frigorific process has been attended with manifest advantage in recent cases of gout and rheumatism, or in such cases as are evidently accompanied with vigorous action and inflammation of sthenic character. In no one of the cases in which this treatment has been pursued, have any ill consequences succeeded to my knowledge; yet those certainly cannot be considered as sufficient evidence to prove its validity in all cases, but sufficient to warrant a continuance of the experiment in all cases of the above description.

" A surgeon of considerable practice in this metropolis, a man of real professional ability, who has been a martyr to the pain and confinement of gout, is continually in the habit of arresting its progress, when he has an opportunity of performing it sufficiently early, by a practice of the kind. When he perceives the
approach

approach of his enemy, he goes to the Thames, and making bare his legs and feet, immerses them in the river from the side of a boat, in which he is rowed about for a considerable time, which seldom fails of producing the effect required. Several cases which have come to my knowledge, in which the feet have in the commencement of an attack of gout been accidentally exposed to cold and moisture, with great advantage, farther tend to justify the belief, that such treatment will in a great variety of cases prove beneficial; though, from the contrary nature of its operation to the plan which has for the most part been hitherto adopted, it is probable that much time must elapse before the remedy can become general *.

" *Jermyn Street,*   " J. RICARDS."
  St. James's.

Cases

* These remarks on the topical application of cold in gouty affection, are highly judicious; they at once view the subject in a guarded light, and discover a liberal desire for the promotion of medical science. The ingenious author has perhaps but too truly predicted that the general adoption of the remedy will not be at a very early period. He knows too well the inveteracy of popular prejudice, not to perceive the difficulty of speedily effecting a revolution in the public mind, in favour of a treatment diametrically opposite to that which has been hitherto admitted and espoused. Though this *slow-paced* correction of habitual

Cases of the curative Efficacy of topical Cold in gouty and rheumatic Affection, communicated by Mr. Custance, Surgeon.

" *To Dr. Kinglake.*

"Sir,

"I was exceedingly gratified on reading your very ingenious paper on the cure of arthritis, inserted in the last number of the Medical and Physical Journal, particularly as it contained the same sentiments on the subject, as I have long entertained in my own mind. I confess I was a long time shackled with *old* opinions, and found it very difficult to adopt the noble declaration of Horace,

"Nullius addictus jurare in verba magistri;"

still more to venture on the trial of a new mode of treating gout.

" However, at length, I made the experiment *last August*; when, being called to a Mr. H.

error is greatly to be deplored, yet the decided efficacy of the refrigerant treatment in promptly extinguishing gouty inflammation, in protecting the constitution from morbid sympathy, in annulling it when existing, and in obviating a useless demolition of systematic strength, is so striking, that a well-founded hope may be indulged, of mankind not being able long to resist a remedy recommended by advantages so vast and glaring.   K.

who

who had resided many years in Jamaica, I found
him attacked with gout, for the second time, in
both great toes. The redness and pain were great,
and the skin was smooth and shining. I directed
a strong solution of sal ammon. c. to be constantly applied, with folds of linen, to the affected
parts, kept his body open with kali tartarisatum,
and occasionally gave an opiate. He pursued
the plan, and was quite well at the end of a
fortnight. This is the only case in which I have
made trial of the plan; but if in any future
communications to the public you should think
this single testimony will corroborate your own
evidence on the subject, you are at liberty to
make what use you please of it.

"I have the honour to be, &c.

"G. CUSTANCE, Surgeon."

"Kidderminster,
December 5, 1801.

"To Dr. Kinglake.

"Sir,

"I duly received your favour of the 25th of
December 1801; and, in compliance with your
request, I have the pleasure to acquaint you,
that I have lately been successful in three cases
of rheumatic fever, by the application of cold to

the parts that were swelled and inflamed. The form I used was half an ounce of sal ammon. c. dissolved in one pint of water. Rags well soaked in this solution were kept constantly to the parts, and the patients expressed their surprise at the ease they experienced from the application, and the good effects were soon visible in reducing the swelling and inflammation. I am now so fully convinced of the perfect safety and utility of the application of cold to rheumatic and arthritic inflammation, that I shall never in future hesitate to recommend it. I had intended communicating my thoughts on the subject to the Editors of the Medical and Physical Journal; but supposing you have it in contemplation to favour the public, in some shape or other, with your own observations, I prefer giving a statement of simple facts to you, which you are welcome to make what use of you judge proper *.

"I am, &c.

"*Kidderminster,*   "G. CUSTANCE."
April 15, 1802.

Case

---

* These cases are strongly in proof of the direct curative power of topical cold in gouty inflammation, The trials were fairly conducted, and the results are demonstrative evidence in its favour. It may be presumed the judicious author used an

ammoniacal

Case communicated by Mr. Dennet to Dr. Kinglake.

"Sir,

"Your former publication, respecting the use of cold water in the gout, excited my attention, and I have often mentioned my ideas of the beneficial effects to be expected from it; but could never induce any patient to adopt the plan.

"The account in the 48th number of the Medical and Physical Journal, determined me (as I had an opportunity) to put it into practice; and though I have but a solitary case to communicate, yet the success was so superior to any other treatment I have seen employed, that I feel it my duty to state it to you. You may make whatever use of it you think proper. I doubt not, you will receive many successful accounts and congratulations from your medical brethren.

"I am, SIR,

"Your obliged humble servant,

"C. DENNETT."

"*Soho Square,*
March 8, 1803.

---

ammoniacal solution more for the convenience of *disguise*, than with a view to any medicinal power it possesses. He, therefore, correctly ascribes its beneficial influence to its coldness, to which indeed it was exclusively due. Simple water is equally, perhaps more, efficient, in as far as it has no stimulant quality.　　K.

" On the third of last month I was requested to visit Mr. Heath, of College Street, Westminster (a carpenter by trade), about forty years of age. The account he gave was, that about a fortnight before he had overheated himself, and afterwards stood in the cold. In a day or two, after this he was seized with shivering and pain in the limbs. The second day the great toe of one foot began to swell, and the ankle was much inflamed. The day after, the other foot and ankle had the same appearance.

" After continuing in this state for three or four days (in which time he had done nothing but applied some spirituous embrocation, as he declined sending for medical assistance, never before having known a day's illness), the complaint shifted to the hands, and then again to the feet. When I first saw him, the feet and ankles were most affected, but he could neither move hand nor foot to assist himself. The efflorescence had every appearance of gout; pulse 120. I was informed by his mother that he had cried out with pain like a woman in labour.

" This case, by nosologists, may be considered as rheumatic gout, but to me the inflammatory excitement is the same. I began my treatment by by ordering the affected parts to be constantly kept wet by cold water; and, that I might ensure due attention to the plan, I sent spring water simply coloured with coccinella, and gave as medicine tinctura opii camphorata, and tinctura guaiaci ammoniata, every four hours. On the fourth, found him easier, the inflammation a little subsided; pulse 100, and full; perspiration all over him; the pain had been very severe in the night; medicine continued. Fifth, much easier; inflammation going off; the bowels being constipated, gave him a dose of pulvis scammonii compositus, et pulvis guaiaci. Seventh, the pain little; efflorescence nearly gone; pulse 80; medicine as before. Ninth, mended in every respect; can move his feet quite easily; sat up two hours. Tenth, inflammation quite gone; has no pain; feels only debility; pulse natural; appetite returned. Twelfth, gave him cinchona, which he continued to the nineteenth, when I took my leave, as he had walked out several times, and found himself perfectly recovered *.

"C. DENNETT."

"Soho Square,
March 8, 1803. Cases

---

* This case affords valuable testimony in support of the cooling treatment in gouty affection. It was adopted with unprejudiced

Cases communicated by Mr. Bartley, Surgeon, to Dr. Kinglake.

" Sir,

" Impelled by the high opinion I entertain of your philanthropy, and invited by your address, contained in the Medical and Physical Journal for February, I venture to trouble you with two or three cases, wherein the application of cold to parts affected with arthritis and rheumatismus acutus, appeared to have been eminently serviceable.

" The first is a case of rheumatismus acutus, in which I duly observed the antiphlogistic treatment, and applied to the part affected the rubefacients which are commonly in use, as linimentum camphoræ compositum, &c.; but so far from any benefit accruing to my patient from the plan, the pain became hourly more intense, although some abatement took place of the febrile symptoms. Thus circumstanced, I was determined to pursue your mode of topical application,

prejudiced confidence, and was, as usual, productive of the desired effect. How very different would have been the situation of this patient in the common mode of practice! His suffering, and consequent debility, instead of continuing but a few days, would have been probably lengthened to as many weeks.   K.

and

and ordered the inflamed parts to be constantly wetted with a mixture of vinegar and water (the former I use to prevent giving alarm to the patient's friends). The good effects were soon perceivable. On the first application of the cloths, which I had directed to be wetted, and changed as often as they became warm, they dried as fast as if held before a large fire; butthe swelling, inflammation, and pain, soon abated, and he enjoyed, on the succeeding night, comfortable sleep, which he had not done for many nights before, owing to the acuteness of the pain. In short, every unpleasant symptom quickly dispersed, and in the space of two or three days he was restored to the enjoyment of health and ease.

" The second case is in the same class with the first, but the attack was much more violent. It occurred in a young subject, of the sanguine temperament. The heat and irritability were excessively great, particularly in the parts affected, which were the ankle joints. Before I was applied to, she was delirious with excess of pain; even the bed-clothes coming in contact with the inflamed parts, would occasion her to scream violently; and she was unable to express the extent of her misery, otherwise than by continual groans. There were considerable tension and swelling

swelling in the parts. I immediately proceeded in the plan which I had before adopted. The relief was instantaneous; pain, swelling, and inflammation, presently subsided; and to the astonishment of her friends the disease retreated as fast as it had advanced: she soon became convalescent.

" The third case is of a gentleman, who having a few days since experienced an unusually violent attack of arthritis, applied to me for relief. He appeared to be particularly averse to any topical application, but the usual one of abundance of flannel. I knew well I should in vain endeavour to persuade him to the application of cold water; prejudices were too strong against me; but I at length prevailed on him that I might be permitted to send him an embrocation, which I assured him he would find highly beneficial. I consequently sent him a quart bottle of water, having put in it about an ounce of spiritus vini camphoratus to give it a smell, and a little of tinctura coccinellæ for the sake of colour, directing that the part might be copiously bathed. He was astonished at its speedy effect, declared it was miraculous, and congratulated me on being in possession of a remedy so valuable for a disease so dreadful. To be brief:

brief: although the pain, swelling, and inflammation were very great, and the parts utterly incapable of motion, yet the next day he was able to walk in his garden, without the assistance of crutches, and is now as well as usual, without having experienced the least return of his complaint.

"If these testimonies which I have thus incoherently stated, may be of service in the promotion of your useful practice, you are at liberty to make what use you please of them.

"With the most ardent wishes for your success in every undertaking, permit me to subscribe myself, with respect*,

"Yours, &c.

"Nailsworth,   "O. W. BARTLEY,
Gloucesteshire,   "Surgeon."
March 9th, 1803.

* The most incredulous, even the most obstinately prejudiced, must admit that these cases decidedly prove the speedy and salutary influence of topical cold in gouty inflammation. Additional evidence might indeed extend the demonstration of its utility, but could not improve its incontestable clearness.   K.

Cases communicated by Dr. Hall.

" To Dr. Kinglake.

" Dear Sir,

" On the appearance of your paper on the subject of gout, in the Medical and Physical Journal for November 1801, it was my intention, had I not been prevented by a severe and tedious indisposition, to transmit you a case which accidentally fell under my own observation; and which in my opinion tends strongly to corroborate the doctrine advanced in that communication, and the safety of the practice therein recommended.

" A few years ago, previously to my leaving Roxburghshire, I was occasionally called, in the exercise of my professional avocations, to visit the family of Mr. Stonehouse, an officer of the excise, residing in Jedburgh. His mother Mrs. Stonehouse, who was at that time considerably upwards of eighty, had been for many years subjected to the frequent recurrence of podagral inflammation, which affected the toes and ankles of both feet. Solely actuated by her own feelings, she perhaps carried the refrigerating plan of treatment to a greater extent than has been hitherto done in the case

of any other patient whatever; as, immediately
on the pain and inflammation becoming troublesome, she plunged the affected limbs into cold
water, which was occasionally renewed, keeping
them immersed in it during the whole day. At
night her bed was adjusted in such a manner as
to expose her limbs to the external air, and she
had water placed by it, so that, on a recurrence
of any painful sensation, she might have recourse to her favourite remedy, without disturbing the rest of the family.

" So fully sensible was she indeed of the benefit to be derived from cold, that even after the
diminution of the pain and heat rendered the
employment of the water no longer necessary,
she used to walk about the house during the most
inclement weather, without either shoes or stockings, notwithstanding the earnest remonstrance
of a very affectionate son and daughter. Mrs.
Stenhouse never had occasion to call in medical
aid, or to have recourse to any internal medicine
whatever; yet, so far from experiencing the
slightest inconvenience, or suffering the least
injury from the liberal use of cold water, on the
contrary, by means of this practice, the violence
of the inflammation and pain was never allowed
to proceed to that degree, as either to impair the

R   vigour

vigour and mobility of the affected parts, or to produce those symptoms of morbid irritation, which are in similar cases so very frequently propagated, by associated influence, over the whole system.

"From repeatedly witnessing the beneficial effects of cold application in the case of this patient, joined with analogical reasoning, I was led to entertain sentiments not essentially different from your own, although a variety of circumstances which it would be here wholly unimportant to relate, prevented me from bringing the practice to the test of farther experiment. Doubtless many other arthritic patients like Mrs. Stenhouse, acting in conformity to their own feelings, and unfettered by prejudice and theories, may have experienced relief from similar means, although, from the circumstances under which such cases occurred, they must necessarily be lost to the public. In illustration of this conjecture, permit me to mention a circumstance recorded in the works of the late Lord Orford, respecting the consort of George the Second, who being in the daily habit, while at Richmond, of walking several miles with him, oftener than once, when labouring under the gout in her foot, dipped the affected limb into cold water, to enable her to attend his Majesty.

"An

"An imperfeet acquaintance with the pathology of gout, and the prejudice very generally entertained respecting the salutary nature of this disease, have, I am fully aware, operated on the majority of practitioners, to represent the effects of cold applications as highly injurious, and as frequently tending to superinduce palsy, apoplexy, and other similar affections; though it should seem much more consonant to fact and observation to consider such morbid effects as the result of a particular state of the system induced by the arthritic diathesis, than as the consequence of employing topical cold, or other analogous remedies. Independently, however, of all hypothesis, the facts you have brought forward in support of the efficacy of reduced temperature in arthritic inflammation, appear to me extremely interesting, and sufficiently marked to warrant the conclusions that have been drawn from them.

"But as the subject is confessedly of great importance, and as the opinion you have attempted to establish militates against that held by persons of great professional respectability, a more enlarged and comprehensive induction of facts may perhaps be necessary in order still farther to confirm the evidence adduced in the

detail

detail of the different cases, in which the mode of treatment has been employed.

" The zeal which you have displayed on the present, as well as on many former occasions, for the improvement of the healing art, will, I trust, communicate itself to the faculty at large, and induce them to co-operate in promoting the accomplishment of the plan you have in contemplation, for establishing the power of topical refrigeration in the cure of arthritic inflammation, on the solid basis of experience and observation.

" Unfortunately indeed for the true interests of science, it too frequently happens that those who dare to think for themselves, and who presume to call in question the truth of doctrines generally received, however fanciful or ill-founded, instead of experiencing that candour and moderation, which should ever be exercised in scientific researches, have met with treatment the most illiberal and absurd. But I flatter myself, however much the practice under consideration may be condemned by individuals whose disposition is to vilify whatever accords not with their own preconceived opinions, that if reason, and not authority, facts and not prescription, be to decide

the

the question at issue, the result will afford a mass of evidence sufficient to convince the most sceptical of the utility of the means you have promulgated for the alleviation of one of the most grievous maladies that can afflict man-kind *.

" I remain,

" Church Row,   " Dear Sir,.
 Hampstead.   " Yours, &c.

June 20th, 1803.   " R. HALL, M. D."

---

* This very intelligent communication is replete with both scientific and practical worth. Its judicious author views the subject with true philosophical criticism and dignified liberality. The case recited valuably applies in refutation of a gratuitous opinion, that topical cold in gouty inflammation is *peculiarly* dangerous in old people, in whom it has been alleged, the powers of life are at too low an ebb to withstand the noxious effects of repulsion. This instance, in addition to many others, controverts that groundless dread, and, in *fact*, authorizes the principle advanced in the preceding work, that the aged, the weak, and morbidly excitable, are *peculiarly* protected, by an early cure of gout, from the various sympathetic evils its protraction threatens ; and that in their case, as in every other, speedy relief from gouty torture is not *repulsion*, but *expulsion*, or annihilation of the disease.   K.

Case communicated by Mr. Nagle.

" *To Dr. Kinglake.*

" Sir,

" Observing in one of the late Medical Reviews, that you solicited medical men to acquaint you with the result of their practice in *your novel remedy* for the gout, has induced me to write to you.

" Mr. Crispin, carpenter of this ship, aged fifty-three, has been subject to the gout for many years, to two or three attacks at least in the course of a twelvemonth, and has been confined for weeks to his cabin, being unable to attend to the duty of the ship. Ten days ago he had a severe attack of gout in the right foot and great toe, which was attended with great pain and inflammation. I ordered him immediately to keep constantly cloths wetted in cold water to the foot, which he was reluctantly persuaded to do, from being always advised before to keep well wrapped up in flannel. To my astonishment as well as his own, in the course of two days every unpleasant symptom left him, and he was able to walk about the ship without a crutch. Leave was given him to go on shore at this place for three days; and on his coming on board, he acquainted me that he went into the salt water daily, supposing

2   in

in his own mind, that a general immersion would be of service to him, from having experienced the good effects of the local application of cold water.

"I am happy to think that *no ill* effect has proceeded from *his temerity*, as it surely was going very far.

"This is the first opportunity in my practice that has occurred of using cold water, as, in talking with many gouty people on the subject, they seem to shudder at the idea, and are afraid of the gout attacking the stomach. If I may judge from this case, and those you have favoured the world with, I have no doubt but it will be attended with inestimable benefit, such as the good effects of cold affusion in fever, which are incalculable according to Dr. Currie's plan *.

"I have the honour to be, &c.

"LUKE F. NAGLE."

*" H. M. Ship Royal Sovereign, ·
Cawsand Bay, Plymouth Dock,
July 24th, 1803.*

* This case would have been exceedingly strong had it stood alone; but perfectly concurring with many similar instances of success adduced in this Appendix, its authority is irresistible. K.

Case

" *To Dr. Kinglake.*

" Sir,

" Your learned elucidation of reduced temperature, which appeared sometime since in the Medical and Physical Journal, I trust will not go unnoticed by even every common observer.

" In justice to your merits in the practice, and to the scientific manner in which it is directed, I beg leave to inform you of a few cases within my own practice, wherein it has been strikingly useful.

" Soon after your first paper appeared in the Medical Journal, my assistant visited a man in acute rheumatism: he had severe pain and swellings in his ankles. Aq. veget. min. was ordered to be applied to the painful parts; the pain the next day shifted to his knees; it was followed with the cold application, and with the same relief. On the third day, when I saw him, he was sitting on a low chair, with a pan of water on each side of him, in which each elbow was rested, which he observed was the only mode of
obtaining

obtaining relief. The man has been before attacked several times with the same complaint, but was sooner relieved this time than under any former practice.

" George Sneath, aged thirty-two, was admitted on the 9th of September, in a regular fit of the gout. He was attacked in the middle of the preceding night with an excruciating pain in the great toe. When I saw him the next morning, his toe and foot were much swollen, and extremely tender. I ordered him an aperient, some four grain doses of Pulv. antim. and the Aq. veget. min. to be applied constantly to the part affected. The man felt much surprised at my treatment, it being so different from the practice he had before used ; but my having attended all his relatives in various situations, I prevailed on him without much trouble to follow my directions, and on the 1st of October he returned thanks to the Dispensary, seemingly much gratified for the benefit he had received, observing that he never before got well half so soon, or with so little pain ; nor did he ever before find himself so little impaired in his general health as at this time.

" I was

"I was met the other day by a benevolent gentleman (with whom this city abounds), who was sympathizing in the fate of a workman of his, who like himself was frequently afflicted with that incurable disorder the gout. He took me to see him, when I told the man that science, aided by Providence, had directed means for his relief, which he earnestly entreated, as the support of his family solely depended on his hard labour. I pursued the same means as in the other case, which terminated very shortly in a cure, much to the satisfaction of the patient, his master, and myself.

"Similar instances I have no doubt will soon follow. Use these as you please, and accept my most sincere wishes for the prosecution of your valuable discovery *.

"I am, Sir,

"Bristol Dispensary,   "Yours respectfully,
October 17th, 1803.   "W. D. ROLFE."

* The refrigerant treatment of gout derives support from these cases; they also evince with what advantage the practice may be adopted in public hospitals, and other medical institutions; but before this desirable benefit can be *extensively* realized, philosophical science and liberality must gain the ascendency of professional routine and prejudice.   K.

Communication

Communication by Mr. Garnsey, Surgeon.

"*To Dr. Kinglake.*

"Dear Sir,

"I feel myself highly obliged to you for your excellent plan of cold application in gout. I can truly say that I have experienced the most happy effects from it. Twenty years ago, when I first felt arthritic affection, I covered the inflamed parts with the warmest flannel I could procure, which kept up such an increased temperature, and left such debility, that I had scarcely recovered of one attack before I had another. When I was first advised by you to pursue a contrary treatment, I had my fears in adopting it, judging it extremely hazardous to repel arthritic inflammation.

"I first began with disrobing the highly inflamed parts of the cumbrous load of flannel, with which they had been usually covered: this reduced in a great degree the morbid heat, so that my fits were not so violent as before. On the next attack (thinking life not worth preserving under such acute pain) I immediately immersed the parts in cold water, which in a few hours carried off the inflammation, so that

I had

I had the use of the limb again in a few days. It was common for me to be confined to a warm room in gout, in most profuse perspiration, for several weeks, and to be so debilitated when the arthritic affection had left me, that I could not stand for a fortnight; but since I adopted the cold plan, I feel such a quick transition from pain to ease, that it scarcely deserves the name of gout.

"I can now walk better than I could ten years ago, which my friends indeed frequently remark; and as I purpose having recourse to the cold bath every morning, I anticipate the pleasing prospect of fully regaining my former pedestrian alertness *.

" I am,

" Dear Sir,

" *North Curry*,   " Yours very sincerely,
January 18*th*, 1804.   " R. W. GARNSEY."

Case

* The instance of the beneficial effects of topical cold here detailed, may be considered as an authority for its adoption in cases of hereditary, long standing, and increasing gout. The disease in this patient, to my own knowledge, occurred early, was

probably

Case and Observations communicated by Mr. Montagu.

" To Dr. Kinglake.

" Sir,

" As Englishmen, I hope we shall ever watch the liberty of the press with the most scrupulous jealousy, as by that privilege the community derive advantages which are highly beneficial. Public prints of public institutions tend to inform and enlighten the age ; and, as such, I am a strong advocate and friend to their existence.

" Philosophy has been many ages emerging from chaotic darkness, and has by no means yet received that light which ought to be expected, nor will it while theory is preferred to practice, for it too frequently happens that philosophers adopt an opinion, and reason thereon, without knowing whether the basis is good, or the

probably of maternal descent, and returned at short intervals, often with extreme violence and long continuance. The cooling treatment (as stated) has so limited the force of its attack and duration, as to have rendered it an ailment of no comparative importance, to what it was, under the exasperating influence of the usual stimulating management. K.

foundation

foundation sound, on which the fabric is erected. Experimental reasoning is the surest guide to truth and sound philosophy; but unfortunately the mind of man receives false impressions, which become rooted by age, and is the ground of continued darkness.

"In perusing various periodical publications in a fit of the gout, I fortunately stumbled upon the number of the Medical Journal, in which were some practical hints of yours upon arthritis, and which so clearly evinced the advantage of the topical application of cold water, supported by experiment and sound reasoning, that I had no hesitation in giving it a trial on myself; and as an account of the method I pursued, and the result, may possibly strengthen the cause in which you are so laudably engaged, and help to eradicate the prejudices under which your discovery will for a time labour, I trust the following will not be unacceptable to you.

"In the latter end of November last I was attacked with the gout in my left foot; the first paroxysm was confined to the second joint of the great toe, and the second extended the inflammation and swelling over the whole of the foot, the outside of which became so painful
that

that no position gave it relief. In this state I directed a poultice made of milk and barley meal, with a little yeast and sweet oil, to be applied when I went to bed *. The pain however continued at night; and though the paroxysm was somewhat abated, I could not put my foot to the ground.

" In this situation, when I expected other paroxysms (my usual lot), and with symptoms of gouty affection in the other foot, which had not escaped its share for some years past, I observed in the aforementioned periodical publication your essay. The poultice was now removed, and I washed off the remainder of it with cold water, and continued wet cloths round my foot for ten minutes or a quarter of an hour, by which time my foot became perfectly easy, and in an hour or two after I was enabled to walk with ease across the room, without the help of a stick.

" The other foot had also been washed with cold water, and the symptoms abated. In this

* A recipe frequently before tried, and was thought to be of service, particularly to the regenerating of strength in the affected parts.

delightful

delightful remission of pain, I continued all day, and at night applied the wet cloths as before, in order to brace and reduce the swelling. The next morning my foot had very little remains of swelling, the same course was observed that morning and night; but about six o'clock the following morning I awoke with some pain in the same great toe; but as it was not materially bad, and at an inconvenient time, I kept removing my foot to all the cold parts of the bed I could find, by which means I kept the part cool, and free from much inflammation, until I arose between seven and eight o'clock, when the cold water application, as before, stopped effectually its farther progress; for I have no doubt, if I had as usual wrapped in flannel, and kept the part warm, two or three paroxysms more would have ensued according to custom.

" From this time no more symptoms of gout occurred, and I continued not only the cold application by cloths, but immersion in cold water, and in the course of three days after, my foot had recovered so much strength, that, had the weather been favourable, I could have taken foot exercise out of doors. Before a week had elapsed, my usual shoe was on, and I walked nearly as well as ever.

" Now,

Now, Sir, I have only to add to this account, that I have been subject to this dreadful disorder more or less these twenty years, usually to one fit in the year during that time, excepting two or three years together at one period.

" My spare make, and active habits, as well as excessive temperance in diet, should not seem to induce inflammation. Plain animal food, cold water, and two glasses of wine, are my usual repast at dinner, and that with a party; the accustomed breakfast, and no call for supper, except a little milk and a crust of bread : with me therefore gout is not the fruit of indulgence.

" Before I conclude this, it may not be amiss to state, that through prejudice from medical opinion, I had long been deterred from the application of cold water, though I had always been inclined to view the disease as you do, and to treat it as a local inflammation, by any application that would quickly carry off the super-abundant accumulated heat, which is apparent in the affected part; to do which, æther perhaps would be infinitely better than any other fluid, from its propensity to evaporate *. Giving way however

* The rapidly evaporant quality of æther at the human animal temperature, renders it undoubtedly refrigerant; but certainly

s   not

however to the reasoning of the profession, I have submitted to much pain and torture, and was always left infinitely worse in health after a fit than before; whereas now, by its short duration, I am, thank God, perfectly well *.

" The first attack of gout I ever had, was when I was about twenty-five years old; it produced but little inflammation or swelling in my foot, but kept me lame for two or three months. Being a keen sportsman, and greatly distressed at my inability to walk at the approach of the shooting season, I arose on the 1st of September, at four

---

not in the degree in which water at the atmospheric temperature operates, and which is requisite to the speedy and effectual extinction of gouty inflammation. The reason is obvious: æther is already surcharged with heat or repulsive motion, and is consequently too fugitive to admit of any considerable addition of that property, previously to evaporating; on the contrary, the comparatively low temperature of cold water, will copiously receive and proportionately transfer inflammatory heat from the affected part. K.

* This is correctly connecting cause with effect. The short duration of local torture prevented the system from being overwhelmed, and permanently distempered by morbid sympathies, which are necessarily in the train of protracted gout, and which may be (as in this instance) invariably obviated by its early cure. K.

o'clock

o'clock in the morning, plunged my foot into cold water, walked the whole day in wet shoes, occasionally putting my foot into a pool of water, and became after it almost instantaneously cured of a lameness that had baffled good medical assistance.

"This ought to have opened my eyes; but prejudice, that bane of improvement, instilled into the mind by others on whose judgment one is apt to place confidence, had kept me blind, and tormented by that dreadful complaint, for which I have no doubt the world as well as myself will in time thank you for the discovery of a remedy, which will make posterity as regardless of its attack, as those who have been vaccinated are at that of the small-pox; for it signifies very little the return of a disorder from the same predisposed state of the animal economy, if a remedy is found for instantaneous cure.

" I shall now conclude by wishing you every success in your farther experiments, against all the mass of opposition you must expect from the old school; but by perseverance, I hope I shall live to see such prejudice done away,

for

for facts are stubborn and incontrovertible things *.

        " I remain, Sir,

" *Knowle House,*   " Your much obliged servant,
Kingsbridge, Devon,   " G. Montagu."
January 14*th*, 1804.

---

* This communication discovers much scientific liberality and public benevolence. It also presents a strong instance of habitual gout promptly yielding to topical refrigeration, with a manifest advantage to the general health. This circumstance indeed is so necessary a consequence, that it would not be adverted to, but for the purpose of additionally refuting the chimerical notion of distant injury being entailed on the constitution, by speedily subduing gouty excitement. This opinion is as extravagant as groundless, as fearful as incomprehensible. It originated at a period when all diseases were supposed to be generated by noxious humours, and when the system was farcically invested with a selective power to detach and remove from the circulating fluids, whatever was *materially* offensive to health. Although this was taking for granted what was *confessedly* too absurd to attempt to prove, yet the phantom has inconceivably kept its ground, and has been at once more or less the *ignis fatuus* of medical practitioners, and the *hobgoblin* of the deluded public, from remote antiquity to the present time.   K.

Case communicated by Mr. Toller.

"*To Dr. Kinglake.*

"Dear Sir,

"It is certainly true that since I was favoured with your advice, I have adopted the cooling treatment when attacked by the gout, and that the effect was attended with all the advantages which the most sanguine supporters of the system could possibly predict. The experiment probably may not be deemed decisive, because the inflammation was slight and in its incipient state.

"I shall readily state to you the particulars of my case, and have not the least objection to their being communicated to the public.

"You will undoubtedly recollect, that I have been subject to the gout during the last fifteen years, and that the paroxysms have been frequent, long, and severe. About a month since I was attacked by a gouty inflammation in my foot, attended with such symptoms as led me to apprehend, that I should be oppressed with a fit of no ordinary duration or severity. I immediately ordered a bucket of cold water, and plunged

s 3　　　　　　　　　　my

my foot into it, and continued it there about twenty minutes. I repeated the remedy four times during the course of the day. The inflammation was checked, but not entirely removed. The next morning I again plunged the disordered foot into cold water, and after repeating the experiment once more, the inflammation and every other menacing symptom were completely removed. But the circumstance which I conceive to be of the utmost importance in my case is this, that, in opposition to the general opinion or prejudice on the subject, I have never felt the least unpleasant sensation in my head or stomach, in consequence of the new treatment to which I have submitted. Yet I must acknowledge that the warm remonstrances of a great number of valuable friends, for whose opinions on other subjects I have great respect, lead me to apprehend some danger from the remote consequences of the new practice *.

"I am,

"*South Petherton,*   "Dear Sir, &c.

February 16*th,* 1804.   " RICHARD TOLEER."

Cases

---

* This case is furnished by a gentleman of distinguished liberality, discernment, and correctness. The result of the
treatment

Cases communicated by Mr. Woodforde, Surgeon.

" To Dr. Kinglake.

" Dear Sir,

" In answer to your note which I had this morning the honour to receive, I beg leave to inform you that from the observations I have made

treatment recited was perfectly decisive, as to its salutary efficacy, in the most desirable manner in which it can be realized, that of arresting the progress of the affection, and thereby preventing the eventual violence to which it would attain, if suffered to proceed unchecked. Had the inflammation been fully formed, the treatment would have been (if possible) still more brilliantly successful. The agonizing torture of high inflammation would then have been almost instantaneously allayed, and consequently have afforded a degree of both local and general relief, that may be justly considered to be at least a state of rapid convalescence, if not of actual cure. This case (it is ardently hoped, and may be as confidently presumed) will ultimately afford all the evidence that even the most visionary apprehension could require, with respect to the *unexceptionable* nature of the cure derived from topical cold in gouty inflammation. The subject of it is yet young, and promises to live long enough fully to satisfy himself, as well as his deservedly anxious friends, that life may be considerably *lengthened* by resisting the destructive tendency of frequent and protracted gout; but that it is physically impossible that it should be either *annoyed*, or abridged, by counteracting the immediate and distant influence of that threatening disease.   K.

on the refrigerant mode of treating gout and inflammatory rheumatism, I have not the smallest doubt in my mind of its salutary effects; and had you not requested my opinion upon it, I should most certainly, from motives of humanity, have considered it as my duty to promote its practice as much as possible. Your present situation enables you to know 1 must have had a very considerable number of patients under my care; and I can with truth assert that in no one instance have I known the mode of treatment fail, or have I witnessed a solitary proof of bad effects resulting from it *,

" I am

* It cannot but be highly gratifying to an honest zeal for the practical improvement of medicine, to learn from such testimony as is here recorded, that not a ' solitary proof ' has occurred of topical cold in gouty affection having been injurious. This favourable experience of its efficacy is the counterpart of my own, and will become that of every unprejudiced observer who will dispassionately regard the authority of fact, and not be misled by preconceived notions and hearsay reports to its disadvantage.

Physical necessity is an immutable operation of nature; and where it obtains, no external opposition can prevail against it. The doctrine of temperature applied to the cure of gout, is of this incontrovertible description. It therefore confidently challenges the adversaries of the practice it inculcates, to adduce a *single instance* of its having ever proved hurtful. Hundreds
may,

"I am well aware you need not the aid of cases to confirm the utility of the practice; but if you should consider the annexed worth your attention, you will of course make what use of them you may think proper.

"I am,

"*Taunton,*   " Dear Sir, &c.

February 20*th*, 1804.   "T. WOODFORDE."

CASE I.

"A young lady, about twenty years of age, was, towards the end of October last, attacked with rheumatic fever; some days had elapsed before I was called to her assistance. I found her labouring under the most severe rheumatic affection I ever witnessed in the course of my practice; her pulse at a hundred and twenty, all the extremities tumefied, with high inflammation, and

---

may, and have been vaguely stated; but *not one* that ever came to my knowledge, would abide the test of common scrutiny; *not one* but would shrink from examination, with all the confusion, littleness, and inadmissibility that correctly characterize the futile attempt to combat well-substantiated facts by adverse and unfounded rumours, whether originating from the proverbial falsehood of *common fame,* or the incorrigible delusion of *medical bigotry.*   K.

acutely

acutely painful; great difficulty of breathing,
with inexpressible anxiety.

" I immediately directed the refrigerant plan,
and was assured by those around her, that my
directions should be fully carried into execution;
but the novelty of the practice, united with the
dreadful apprehension of repulsion, prevented its
being done at *this* time. The patient living at
some distance from me, I did not see her again
till the following day, when I found her labouring under increased disease, with every alarming
symptom that could attend her. I had then no
alternative, but that of having the application
made in my presence; and I experienced the
gratification of seeing its good effects before I
quitted the room. I directed the plan to be regularly persevered in during the remainder of the
day and night, which was, I believe, strictly attended to. I saw her again the following day,
and found she had had refreshing sleep, the
pulse at ninety, much more free from pain, and
the alarming symptoms subsided. Without
going more into the minutiæ of this case, I have
only to add that the plan was discretionally
pursued for about ten days, all painful sensation
ceased, she gradually recruited her strength, and
is now in perfect health.

                                   " I think

" I think it incumbent on me to say, *this patient owes her existence* to the refrigerant mode of treatment.

CASE II.

" A lady, about thirty-eight, of a very delicate constitution, has for more than twelve years been severely and periodically afflicted with hereditary confirmed gout, to so great a degree, that through the winter months she is confined to her room, and generally to her bed. I have often attended her during her painful confinement, and once witnessed her narrow escape from dissolution.

" In the month of September last I was requested to see her; when I found her with inflamed gout in both hands; the elbows also shared a proportion of the disease, and considerable tumefaction, with acute pain, had taken place. I entreated her to try the cold application; she consented to it, and in a few hours was much relieved. It was the next day repeated; after which the pain and swelling totally subsided, and she continued better than she had been for many months before, till the November following, when she was again attacked. The

The disease had now complete possession of all the extremities, the inflammation was very considerable, and the pain *insufferably acute*. The cold fluid was again incessantly applied to all the limbs, and in the course of the next day I had the satisfaction to find the inflammation and pain considerably lessened, and much more relieved than I had expected from a seizure so severe. The plan was rigidly pursued by those about her person for a few days. She gradually recovered strength without the aid of tonics, and has continued well ever since.

CASE III.

"An old man, between seventy and eighty, subject to periodical gout, was in the month of October last violently seized with it in one of his hands. The inflammation ran high, and the pain was intolerable. Linen cloths made wet with the cold fluid were *twice only* applied : at the end of four days there were no remains of gout, and he has from that period continued to be in perfect health.

"I have to remark in this case, that, had the application of cold been delayed, I have no
doubt

doubt but the patient would have undergone a general attack, and been laid up for several weeks, if not months *.

" *Taunton,*   " T. WOODFORDE."
February 20*th,* 1804.

* These cases are inestimably valuable. They make an irresistible appeal to common sense, and unprejudiced reason, against the idle objections which are held respecting the safety of the anti-inflammant remedy. Here are three instances, detailed with much clearness and unquestionable fidelity, in which the cooling treatment proved eminently salutary, in the most difficult and critical circumstances of rheumatic and gouty affection. If on these several occasions the topical use of diminished heat actually repelled a *remedial disease,* whither did it direct its noxious course? What symptoms discovered its baneful retreat? Has it taken up a dormant residence in the system, or has it not been dissipated to a *nonentity,* by an *expulsive* instead of *repulsive* effect of the treatment? This is the real fact; it is no mystery; it is nothing more nor less than the extinction of inflammatory temperature: and surely the fire that is extinguished has lost its burning quality, and never will spontaneously rekindle. *De nihilo nihil fit.*   K.

Case

Case communicated by Mr. Bancombe, Surgeon.

" *To Dr. Kinglake.*

" **Dear Sir,**

" As it is an object of the greatest importance to those who are unfortunately subject to arthritic complaints, to have the question decided, whether the application of cold in that disease can at all times be admitted, with as much safety to the constitution of the patient, as it is of immediate relief to his sufferings, I send you the following statement of my case, which, if you think will contribute in any degree to so desirable an event, you are at liberty to make any use of you please.

" About six weeks since, I was seized with a smart attack of gout in my right foot (the third time in my life, and within about six years); the disease continued increasing nearly thirty hours, during which I suffered most intolerable pain (particularly in the night), and the part was much swollen and inflamed. In this state I had recourse to cold application, which I used with the greatest freedom by night and day, sometimes

4　　　　　　　　　immersing

immersing the foot into a vessel of cold water, at others wrapping it up in cloths wetted with that fluid, and renewing them as often as they grew warm. This was continued at longer or shorter intervals, as the heat and pain returned, for three days, after which the inflammation and pain being removed, it was discontinued, and by the application of a thin linen bandage, in less than a week I was able to walk about the house.

"In the second night the disease attacked the left ankle severely; but by having recourse to the same remedy the pain was soon relieved, and in a few days all appearance of disease was removed.

"During the use of the cold application, I did not experience the slightest ill effect in the head, stomach, or any other vital organ; and from the present good state of my health, I have no reason to dread any future ill consequence *.

"I am,

"*Taunton*,　　　　　"Dear Sir, &c.

February 5th, 1804.　　　　"J. BANCOMBE."

* This is one among the numerous cases, in which *ocular demonstration* enables me to speak very confidently of the salutary efficacy of topical cold in gouty inflammation. As in every other

other instance, it speedily alleviated the debilitating irritation, which in this painful disease is the *grand desideratum*. The extension of sympathetic mischief to the system, is either restrained, or wholly prevented, by the cessation of local pain. Hence the patient may *truly* say, " no ill effect arose in any of the vital organs." These parts were protected, instead of being either actually embarrassed or endangered by notional repulsion. To entertain dread of future evil from the cure of a disease, is to indulge in a degree of fearful imagination, which *gout alone* (from a strange abuse of custom) countenances; but which is as little sanctioned by correct reason and experience, as it would be were it applied to the most common cases of inflammatory affection, whether from internal or external causes. Thus an inflammation of the brain, lungs, stomach, bowels, or any other vital organ, from either checked perspiration or any other source of morbid excitement; or of the skin, muscle, or bone, from incision, contusion, or fracture, may be as justly said to involve constitutional safety by *early cure* as that of gout; and it would be neither less humane, nor less scientific, to prohibit the immediate relief of those ailments under the dreadful denunciation of *consequent death*, than to forbid promptly remedying gouty disease, which is nothing more than a greater or less degree of inflammatory excitement of the ligamentous and tendinous structure. In spite of the manifold opposition of prejudice, in defiance of all its hostile devices, time will fully elucidate and verify this important position.   K.

Second

Second anonymous Attack*, signed 'Constant Reader,' on Dr. Kinglake's Mode of treating Gout.—Extracted from the Medical and Physical Journal for February 1804.

" To the Editors of the Medical and Physical Journal.

" Gentlemen,

" A temporary absence from home prevented me from seeing the number of your excellent Journal for December last, till it was too late to expect any thing then forwarded could be in‑serted; else the following statement should have reached you earlier.

---

* Although anonymous, this publication is included in this Appendix, to afford me an opportunity of restating my defence against the author's unwarrantable charges. It will be also seen by the perusal of this attack, and by my particular anno‑tations, and general reply to it (the latter of which has been likewise published in the Medical and Physical Journal), how far the Editors of that work have sustained their claim to public confidence as *impartial reporters*, by the renewed and full indul‑gence they have given to the virulent sarcasm of an anonymous writer, who had been confessedly detected in obtruding on the public, through the medium of their Journal, a *hearsay* and *groundless rumour*, for an *authentic fact;* and by the unjustifiable manner in which they have thought fit to mutilate my commu‑nication, by suppressing what might have been justly stated, and adding what obscures and misrepresents my meaning.   K.

" I ac‑

" I acknowledge myself flattered by the honour Dr. Kinglake has conferred on me, by inserting the whole of the observations on cold water a second time.

" It must needs be a good story that will bear being twice told. The anecdote of the late Dr. Gregory I had been in the habit of hearing so frequently repeated, even from my earliest years, by a person entitled to my utmost confidence, and one who was an intimate friend and warm admirer of the liberal mind and manly virtues of the Doctor, that I never even doubted of the truth *.

" Even the Editors of the Annals of Medicine allow, that such a report was prevalent in Edin-

---

* Impartial reader! here pause one moment, and compare this pitiful recantation, with what the author exultingly asserted in his attack. Has he there merely said that a friend entitled to his utmost confidence had frequently repeated to him the anecdote of Dr. Gregory? No; but that this friend *(in propria persona) actually* called on the Doctor, and *found him* bathing his feet in cold water; he then details the remonstrating dialogue that ensued on the occasion, adding, under the authority of this *same friend*, that the Doctor was found in his bed lifeless the next morning. Such a statement, it must be dispassionately allowed, fully warrants the solemn inference, *that either there was no friend in the case, or that he must be an arrant impostor, totally lost to every moral obligation of truth.* K,

.burgh

burgh ' at the time of the Doctor's death, and which has not previously, to my knowledge, been , contradicted.

" Dr. Kinglake's triumph does not seem very complete, even admitting the falsehood of the statement *.

" Nothing more than a negative proof in support of his doctrine can be derived from it, as it only shews that persons of a gouty diathesis are liable to sudden death, even though they do not plunge their extremities in cold water †.

" The reason of my addressing you at present, Gentlemen, is to express my regret at having been the cause of bringing the respected name

---

*" Even admitting the falsehood of the statement." Is it doubted? Has not *peccavi* been *disgracefully*, because *reluctantly* exclaimed? Will the *eye-witnessing friend* again come forward with his *ocular proof*, his *demonstrative evidence* ?   K.

† You are pushed inconveniently hard, 'Constant Reader.' You were but very lately vauntingly dealing in *positive* opposition; and now, oh sad reverse ! flying for shelter in allowing me 'a *negative* proof only' in support of my doctrine. But you say, 'my triumph is not complete.' It is enough that my *negative truth* subdues your *positive falsehood*, to afford me as ample a portion of it as is needful.   K.

of

of the late **Dr.** Gregory into question on so trivial an occasion *; or of occasioning to the present, my much-respected master, the trouble of contradicting the statement.

" My error was truly unintentional †; and I trust Dr. Gregory and his friends will consider this acknowledgment of it as an adequate apology.

" In considering me as hostile to medical im‑ provement, Dr. Kinglake appears evidently to mistake the tendency of my observations.

---

* " On so trivial an occasion." Is an attempt to resist the efficacy of an unparalleled remedy for one of the most deplorable maladies incident to mankind by *falsehood, trivial ?* Or could the venerable memory of Dr. Gregory be more *sacri‑ legiously* treated, than by endeavouring to found a base fabrica‑ tion on his *positive,* his *viva voce authority,* that of his having actually discoursed on the effects of a practice in his own case, which he never adopted ? Truth at once disdains such conduct, and spurns such *guilty* apology.   **K.**

† That is to say, you hoped an assertion convenient to your object, might *perchance* prove true; for which you had no other authority than *hearsay report ;* though you affirmed its veracity to be grounded on the credit of a confidential friend, who, by your account, had been *bona fide* an eye-witness of the fact !!! If this be unintentional error, it is far, *very far* indeed, from *honest* correctness.   `K.`

      " No

"No man, who has taken upon himself the grave important duty of superintending the conduct of his fellow-creatures, during the melancholy visitations of bodily disease, could, I trust, be so deficient in the common duties of humanity, as to neglect or despise any species of information that would tend to mitigate pain, or shorten the duration of misery *. No fault was imputed to Dr. K. for attempting to cure the gout by the application of cold water. The effects of temperature in modifying diseased action, at present attracts much of the attention of the medical world; and when they have been more accurately determined by time and experience †, will, in all probability, extend the dominion of regular science over the functions of the living body.

"To extenuate the spirit of levity and wrangling which Dr. K. has discovered in the tri-

---

* This is downright *hypocritical cant*, in one who officiously and falsely opposed an *idle rumour* against the acknowledged benefits of a practice, as a *fact*, the 'authenticity of which might be depended on.' K.

† And when they shall be less malevolently undermined by 'Constant Reader's' *fabrication* of *adverse facts*, may be justly added. K.

fling

fling * article alluded to, I shall beg his leave
to use the apology employed by Horace on a
similar occasion † :

O! imitatores, servum pecus, ut mihi sæpe,
Bilem, sæpe *jocum* vestri movere tumultus.

" What in truth moved my bile, was the
pompous manner in which Dr. K. announced
the application of cold water in gout, as a novel
practice originating with himself ‡; and for which
he

* Worse than ' *trifling* ;' utterly contemptible, because founded in malicious falsehood. K.

† " On a similar occasion." Horace revered truth, and
never, like this *soi-disant fact-making critic,* prostituted his
satire to malevolent purposes. In these lines the virtuous bard,
with just indignation, lashed the real plagiarist, but never meant
them to be the vehicle of anonymous malignancy ; *a malignancy,*
equally incapable of correctly discriminating, and revengeful
at being discovered in an earnest endeavour to promulgate as an
undoubted truth, a *gross falsehood.* K.

‡ " As a novel practice originating with himself." Where is
the proof of this assertion ? It does not exist. The charge therefore recoils on its author, with apparently a similar indifference
to truth, to that which he has exhibited in the *forged fact* respecting Dr. Gregory's death. My claim to novelty and originality
aspired' much higher than ' Constant Reader' is *willing* to
charge me with, that of conceiving and publishing a doctrine
of

he seemed hastily to solicit the applause due to a public benefactor. A little irony * appeared not ill calculated to repel such an arrogant and unfounded assumption ; but the Doctor, it seems, does not like a joke :

Ludus enim genuit trepidum certamen et iram,
Ira, truces, inimicitias, et funebre bellum †.

---

of gout, which justified the topical application of cold water on sound philosophical principles, regardless of who had been the first casually to have applied the remedy, from a full conviction that its *general use* could never obtain in the existing state of medical, as well as popular prejudices against it, while the practice remained unsanctioned by scientific authority. The remedy indeed was so rarely resorted to, that not a single instance (as already affirmed) was previously known to me, of its having ever been subjected to trial; nor without my *theoretic persuasion* of its perfect safety and salutary efficacy (in which it may be presumed neither 'Constant Reader' nor his group of authorities will pretend to have had any share), should it have been either countenanced or adopted by me for the universe. Have you not then, 'Constant Reader,' as egregiously as malevolently mistaken original and independent thinking for plagiarism ? K.

* " A little irony," well timed, is not amiss; but to adopt the provocation alleged by 'Constant Reader,' not even 'arrogance' and 'assumption' could warrant a single shaft from the *deliberately bent* bow of *falsehood*. K.

† Neither joke nor anger, 'Constant Reader,' has induced my animosity against you. The adeptness you have shewn at fabricating facts adverse to the interests of truth, has *solely* occasioned it.
K.

" With

" With your permission then, Gentlemen, I will proceed to an investigation, more serious and becoming professional gravity and decorum, concerning the validity of the Doctor's claim to originality in the application of cold water to the cure of gout.

" To begin at the beginning, that is, with Hippocrates—Aphorism 25. sect 5. (I need not trouble you with the Greek text) are the following words: " Tumores autem in articulis, et dolores aliisque ulcera, et podagricos, et convulsiones horum plurima, *frigida multa affusa, et levat et attenuat, et dolorem solvit* *. Torpor enim modicus doloris solvendi vim habet." The same doctrine is repeated in nearly similar words in the chapter De Humidorum Usu.

---

* " Et dolorem solvit." Was it ever doubted? Is the character of Hippocrates here exalted by ascribing to him an originality, which had its source in a much remoter age of antiquity than that in which the *Coan* sage lived? He simply states that cold alleviates and subdues pain, which is no more than what ever has, and what ever must be, the *common-place language* of *common-place* sensation. Does either Hippocrates, or any other author, whether ancient or modern, vindicate such alleviation or subduing of pain in gout, by saying, that the affection is merely a local, and not a constitutional disease, and that consequently it has no well-founded claim to be *patiently endured*, as a *remedial grievance?* No; but it is the *boasted originality* of my doctrine to have affirmed the fact, without fear of refutation.   K.

" Among

" Among the remedies recommended by Celsus, ' De Manuum et Pedum Articulorumque Vitiis,' we read as follows : ' Si vero tumor calorque est utiliora sunt refrigerantia, in aqua, quam frigidissima articuli continentur.' Again : ' Levant spongia imposita quæ subinde ex oleo, vel aceto, vel aqua frigidissima exprimitur *.'

" But to come nearer our own times: did the Doctor, in the pursuit of his cold water lucubrations, never stumble on a work by Hermanus van der Heylen, entitled, Aquæ frigidæ inter inauditas, et incredibiles alias Effectus Podagræ · Dolores, vel sistentis, vel mirabiliter demulcentis, et ischiadicos Dolores penitus extirpantis, &c.? From an English translation of this book now lying before me, I shall treat the Doctor with a quotation.

" After shewing very clearly, that pains of the gout are caused either by a hot humour, or by an acrimonious or salt one, proceeding from the liver, Vander exclaims, ' But seeing it is confessed and assented to by all physicians, *that contraries are cured by contraries,* why may I not

* This is no more than the echo of Hippocrates's opinion, in common with that of *human sensation.* K.

lift

lift up my voice, and make use of my pen, in the just praises of this our cold water?' Vander also lays claim to the discovery of the use of cold water, though I do not believe he was ignorant of its having been recommended both by Hippocrates and Celsus, whatever Dr. K. may be. 'But suppose,' says he, 'that the excellent virtues of cold water in the cure of this disease, were never before discovered to the world; or that either its excellencies, in other the like cases, have hitherto been neither written nor heard of; is it impossible to say or write any thing that may be deduced out of the very principles of nature, which may be of good use in curing the diseases men are subject unto, and particularly of the intolerable pains of the gout, and the like? Certainly there are divers that having by experience found the excellent virtue of cold water, for assuaging of those horrid torments of the gout (which are a second hell), will be ready with a very grateful remembrance, publicly to extol the same.' Van clearly deserves the palm for modesty; he only insinuates that he would wish to be considered as the inventor of the cold water system *, but does not absolutely say he is so.   " Smith's

* " Inventor of the cold water system." To what practical benefit could his wish to be considered as the inventor be turned ?

" Smith's Curiosities of common Water, a well-known work, which has passed through many editions, contains abundance of recommendations in favour of the use of cold water in gout, and rheumatism *.

But putting aside these old-fashioned books, has Dr. K. never seen the modern and truly excel-lent treatise of Mr. Rigby on animal heat †? In this

To none at all. The quotation here cited makes him blunder on that *acrimony* or morbid humour, which in all ages, from the remotest antiquity, down even to the present time, has been more or less avowedly held to be the proximate cause of gout, and has consistenly established the prevailing curative indi-cation of inviting rather than checking the offending matter to the gouty part. My doctrine ascribes the disease solely to excessive temperature, considers it as purely local, rejects the nonsense of morbid matter critically deposited from the consti-tution, and consistently directs its cure by the refrigerant in-fluence of rapid evaporation. This *mighty* quotation then, 'Constant Reader,' misses its aim. It exposes your want of correct discrimination, but does not in any shape interfere with my avowed originality. K.

* Does the author justify the practice on principle? If not, its salutary efficacy, however unquestionable, could never gain it public adoption. K.

† This book has never fallen in my way; it has indeed been mentioned to me by a friend, but not until after my commu-nications on gout had been published, when it was my wish that

this work the local application of cold water in the gout, and in various exanthematous complaints, is treated of in a scientific manner *, and illustrated by apposite cases and legitimate deductions.

" In the sixth volume of the Medical Observations, some instances of the utility of cold in the gout, accompanied with many pertinent reflections by the person who was himself the subject

that my view of the subject should proceed as it had begun, wholly uninfluenced by any authority; but for this reason, that publication should have been consulted by me. My friend however, who appeared to be conversant with its merits, gave me not the smallest hint of the author having considered the disease on the principles of the doctrine advanced by me; the work therefore did not interest my originality. With me it can be of no importance when, where, or with whom, the *mechanical practice* of topically applying cold water to gouty inflammation originated; the *ownership* claimed by me is its scientific justification. K.

* " In a scientific manner." The general meaning of this phrase is too vague and indefinite to be adduced in opposition to any particular doctrine that may be the object of attack. How does it trench on my view of the subject ? Does it anticipate my opinion by making gout a disease of excessive temperature, of local origin, and of easy and safe cure? If not, our views of science differ, involve no originality, and prove that 'Constant Reader' is less adroit in critical quotation, than in glossing falsehood with the semblance of truth. K.

subject of the reflections, may be found *. And now, gentlemen, I will leave it with you to determine whether any man, on the revival of a practice which has been so frequently brought forward, and again abandoned (on good grounds or not, Is foreign to the present argument †), be entitled

to

* "May be found." And why not stated? Why are not those 'pertinent reflections' adduced in a way that would directly bear on the question at issue? The fact of cold water alleviating the pain of gouty inflammation, has no essential connexion with the warranty proposed by me for its salutary efficacy as derived from the nature of the disease. This Proteus-like assailant shifts his ground, varies his weapons, charges, retreats, fabricates, and quotes, without ever coming to the point which constitutes the true subject of dispute. Though the use of topical cold in gouty affection might have been recommended from the earliest period of time, and have been resounded through ancient and modern authors, to the present instant, it avails not a tittle against my originality, if no one before me ever *doctrinally* affirmed that gout was a local and not a constitutional disease, that its systematic form was merely a sympathetic diffusion of pain, or motive excitement from the affected part; and consequently the more speedily and effectually the gouty inflammation can be subdued, the more salutary. The application of cold water therefore, abstractedly considered, forms no integrant part of the doctrine; it appeared to me to be at once simple, and of a temperature sufficiently low, curatively to transfer the redundant heat of gouty inflammation. K.

† No; the grounds on which the practice has been taken up, and abandoned, are very essential indeed to the argument. It is

on

to call out *Eureka*, as if he were the first who had passed the pons asinorum.

"Whatever may be the relative merits of the three remedies, the pump, the tincture, and cold water, it must be allowed there was a singular coincidence in their being ushered into public notice about the same time. Nor do I think it shewed any very reprehensible degree of timidity in a man whose daily bread depends on assisting poor human nature, to contend against the gout, and the other various ills that flesh is heir to, to express some degree of alarm at the combined appearance of three remedies, each in its single unaided strength, promising to extirpate a complaint whose existence has in all ages contributed so liberally to the support of every branch of the faculty, and the more so, as it commonly sin-

on the untenableness of former grounds, and the consequent abandonment of the practice, and the tenableness of my grounds and its consequent adoption (or *revival*, if 'Constant Reader' would prefer that term), that my originality is founded, and from which alone a confident, general, and permanent establishment of the remedy could result. You bungle so sadly, 'Constant Reader,' on the most obvious points of discrimination, that you have much less chance of exclaiming 'Eureka' on subjects of criticism, than you appear to have had in passing the 'pons,' not 'asinorum,' but *mendaculorum*.   K.

gles

gles out its victims among the rich and the timid.
Those fears have now indeed in great measure
subsided. Of the pump not much is heard.
The tincture, though, if uncontradicted rumour *
spoke true, supported on the wings of a genius,

Vitreo daturus
Nomina ponto,

is gone to the tomb of all the Capulets, and is
now less heard of, and probably less employed,
than Dr. Solomon's Anti-impetigines. And
though the celebrated Hoffman wrote a treatise
De Aqua Medicina universali, the ravages of disease have not yet ceased to limit the numbers
of mankind; nor do I believe that gout is exter-
minated from the face of the earth †.

" Conscious of having trespassed too long on
your patience, I now take my final leave of Dr.

* Don't be squeamish, 'Constant Reader;' you have fully
proved that whatever may be the quality of a *rumour*, however
improbable it may be, it is still a *raw material* that cannot fail
to issue from your *fact-making manufactory*, as an authentic
truth.   K.

† Nor can it be while such characters as 'Constant Reader'
are malevolently occupied in promulgating as *authentic facts,*
false rumours, adverse to the confident adoption of the only natural and adequate remedy for the evil, namely, *sufficiently*
reduced temperature.   K.

Kinglake,

Kinglake, impressed with a well-founded confidence, that he will in future entertain that kind of friendship and regard for me, which a man generally entertains for another, to whom he feels himself under an obligation *. Dr. K. through the medium of the Medical and Physical Journal, called for materials to assist him in making a book. I have furnished him with some †, and pointed out the pregnant sources of others. The quotations I have inserted, require no other authority than a reference to the books

---

* Not until a disposition to falsehood, equal to that which 'Constant Reader' has manifested, shall have subdued my love of truth, can there be any thing of congeniality or admission of favour, that could lead me to a sense of obligation to that detected and degraded fabricator of *authentic facts*. Such conduct, and such silly exultation, are really far below all contempt. K.

† "I have furnished him with some." You have indeed, 'Constant Reader,' most lamentably for your own credit. My application to the medical fraternity was for correct intelligence; you listened not to the voice of truth; it suited not your malignancy so to do; you officiously obtruded an *unsubstantiated rumour* for an *authentic fact*, hoping thereby to crush at one *deadly blow*, my doctrine and practice in embryo; but your shaft reached not its mark, it fell harmless before the shrine of truth, and served the useful purpose of proclaiming your forfeiture of all future *credibility*. K.

from

from which they are extracted*; I shall, therefore, still request your permission to remain shrouded in my veil of anonymous concealment, as Dr. K. very neatly phrases it. This determination is perhaps less the result of fear of my antagonist, than of a peculiar aversion to medical controversy †.

" Though I will not pledge myself, that when the Doctor shall have published the book with which he has threatened the world, if I do not think his facts well established ‡, and his deductions

---

* The *ipse dixit* of ' Constant Reader,' after the specimen he has given of the low value he sets on truth, would be much too suspicious for my confidence, if it were an object to refer to those authorities; but as the citations which 'Constant Reader' has adduced, as containing their most specious pretences, afford nothing that opposes my argument for originality, my time shall not be misemployed in examining them.   K.

† No, ' Constant Reader,' this was no part of your motive. At least, for *once*, speak the truth ; or if you cannot, allow me to do so for you.   The estimate you placed on your credit in society, *solely* restrained you from hazarding your name to the falsehood your malevolence anonymously obtruded on the public.   K.

‡ You have given ample proof of superior dexterity in fabricating from a *groundless rumour* an *authentic fact;* by the devices of the *same art* you may also display your skill in attempting

u   to

tions logical, I may not start up, *propria persona*, and endeavour, through the aperture of a goose's quill, to throw cold water on the whole *. Till that auspicious æra arrive, I shall continue to regulate my practice in the gout, as I have hitherto endeavoured to do, by the precepts founded on the painful, personal observation of the honest and judicious Sydenham.

" I am, &c.

" A CONSTANT READER."

to transmute my *authentic facts* into *groundless rumours.* But take care lest your *tutelary spell* be again broken, the delusion of your craft be again exposed, and lest repeated failure sink you into the gaping abyss of utter contempt.   K.

* Arrogance and presumption with a vengeance, 'Constant Reader;' but even more licentious vanity might be expected from a 'shrouded' writer like yourself, who entered the list of opposition brandishing the horrible weapon of falsehood. The execution of your threat, however (it may be fairly anticipated), will be as impotent as ridiculous. You will do well to recollect, that whatever you may hereafter advance will be admitted with cautious limitation, from your notoriety in publishing as an *authentic fact* a *groundless rumour*; therefore, both for your own sake, and for the interest of truth, be more scrupulously guarded in what you may hereafter assert, than you have hitherto been.   K.

Dr.

Dr. Kinglake's Reply to 'Constant Reader's' second Attack, published in the Medical and Physical Journal for March 1804.

"To the Editors of the Medical and Physical Journal.

"Gentlemen,

"It is my endeavour to observe as a regulating maxim in my conduct, *Fac nihil per iracundiam*; nor shall my anger even be inordinately excited by the renewed and unprovoked attack of 'Constant Reader,' envenomed as it is with Horatian satire, '*bilious*' acrimony, and *pointless* * wit.

"Such weapons are, in my estimation, never respectable; and, when wielded in the clumsy and misdirected manner of your 'shrouded' correspondent, are *utterly contemptible* †.

* Erroneously printed 'disappointed' in the Medical and Physical Journal, No. 61, p. 241, l. 5.   K.

† For the phrase *utterly contemptible*, are substituted in the Medical and Physical Journal, No. 61, p. 241, l. 8, the words '*more than pointless.*' Is not the legitimate authority of editorship here unwarrantably stretched? The utmost power of that public engagement has always appeared to me to be inviolably restricted to the right of either rejecting a communi-

cation

"My refutation of 'Constant Reader's' mis-
statement was that which truth required; and
the mode in which it was done, had too much
of urbanity either to '*move bile*' or justify
ridicule.

'Tolle jocos, non est jocus esse malignum.'

"My want of triumph, however, is 'Constant
Reader's' exultation. But why this revengeful
satisfaction? Does he regret that the *truth* is
discovered? Was he actuated by either a *sug-
gestio falsi*, or *suppressio veri*, with respect to
the unfounded report? This is indeed a malicious subterfuge, and much too suspicious to be
consistent with the sincere regard he professes
for medical improvement and humanity.

" Although cold water did not destroy in the
instance alluded to; yet as death happened,
destruction, in the opinion of 'Constant Reader,'
must still be in the case, and then this casuistic
declaimer, this faithful reporter of facts, says,
gouty diathesis struck the deadly blow *." Does
he sudden

cation as *inadmissible*, or to report it with *undeviating* fidelity.
Authors surely are entitled to speak for themselves, and should
not be discretionarily misrepresented by Editors.   K.

* The passage included in inverted commas, beginning with
although, and ending with *deadly blow*, was, as nearly as my
recollection

sudden death never happen but from gouty diathesis? Are not the violent and manifold influence of vascular plenitude, obstruction, rup-
ture, and convulsive actions, occurring in the
vital organs, sufficient to account for sudden
death, without gratuitously referring to a ghostly
something, called *gouty diathesis?* The only
diathesis allowable to ' Constant Reader,' on
this occasion, is that of revenge, for having
been detected in attempting to authenticate a
false rumour.

" Has not rancour here usurped the place of
gratitude? and does the *assumed* love of truth

recollection, unaided by correct notes, can serve me, in the original manuscript of my reply, communicated for publication in
the Medical and Physical Journal, but has been as unjustifiably, as
injuriously to my meaning, suppressed by the Editors of that work.
The observation therein contained is pertinently introductory
to 'Constant Reader's' attempt to kill by *gouty diathesis*, when
he had been vanquished in his *cold water* endeavour. Thus to
disjoin the word. *diathesis* from its context, and as abruptly as
inappositely to commence a sentence with it, is at once a barba-
rous mutilation, and a trespass on the perspicuity of the original. The conduct of the Editors, on this occasion, must experience a corrective comment in their own feelings, and in those
of the unbiassed reader, more suitable than may become me to
exhibit. K.

here

here appear unexasperated by the defeat of falsehood?

> " Scelus intra se tacitum qui cogitat ullum,
> Facti crimen habet *."

"In very few words my vindication shall be restated, from all the reproachful, illiberal, and unmanly insinuations of 'Constant Reader,' relative to my claiming an originality in the use of cold water in gout; and then let the public impartially say, what is *offensive cavilling*, and what is an *original* and *honest* endeavour to improve practical medicine. The ground on

---

* The passage designated by inverted commas, beginning with 'Has not,' and ending with '*crimen habet*,' was in the original manuscript of my reply, and has also been suppressed by the Editors of the Medical and Physical Journal. What is the objection to it? It is not in answer to any one who is entitled to gentleness of treatment, but to an anonymous *some person* calling himself 'Constant Reader;' who, after having been detected and exposed in an endeavour to substantiate, in the most suspicious manner, a *groundless report* for an *authentic fact*, was again indulged by the Editors of the Medical and Physical Journal, in assailing me in a style of sarcasm, that *impartial censorship* ought not to have published, without the responsibility of a real signature. But these same Editors have assumed the insufferable liberty of garbling and misrepresenting my reply. 'Constant Reader,' indeed, might have consistently done this, but it was grossly unworthy the public reporters of medical literature. K.

which

which cold water was proposed by me as a safe and effectual remedy for gout, was founded on a radical resemblance which appeared to me to subsist between gouty and every other description of inflammation; that they were also in *common* * of local, and not of constitutional origin; and that, by parity of reason, they ought to yield to similar treatment.

" That this was my view of the subject, is verified by the following quotation from my former reply to 'Constant Reader,' published in the Medical and Physical Journal †.

" It has never been my object to assume credit for either *originality* or peculiarity, in reducing the morbid excess of temperature in arthritic affection by diminished heat. It is impossible the principle should have escaped the earliest reasoning on the subject. The principle of the practice may, therefore, be rather considered as *common* to human intelligence, than *peculiar* to any individual. The doctrine of distempered heat at once pervades and constitutes the most intelligent and instructive

---

* Erroneously printed 'commencement' in the Medical and Physical Journal, No. 61, p. 242, l. 10. K.

† See *first* reply to 'Constant Reader,' republished in this Appendix. K.

parts

parts of Hippocrates's writings. The medical principles and practice of Sydenham, also founded on temperature, formed a transcendent epoch in the history of curative medicine, and, happily for mankind, finally overthrew the fatal delusion of humoral pathology and alexipharmic jargon. Conducted then by analogy, it occurred to me as highly reasonable, that gout, distinguished, like other inflammations, by excessive heat, and marked by no essential difference, might be subdued in a similar manner. This persuasion induced me to assimilate the treatment. Not a single fact had previously reached my knowledge, to authorize the trial; though undoubtedly many were extant. To me therefore the practice was relatively, though not absolutely original. The only claim to originality which seems to exist in my right, and the only one which deserves a moment's solicitude to establish, is that of publicly recommending the practice after experiencing its salutary effects in numerous instances, in which the treatment was conducted with such disguise and secrecy as were necessary to obviate the prohibitive influence of prevailing prejudices against it *."

" The

---

* This is the only claim set up by me for originality in the *practice* of topically applying cold water to gouty inflammation; but

"The shelves of neither ancient nor modern
authors offered any thing that suited the object
of my inquiry. It would be in vain to search
the stores of medical literature for any authority
to countenance my principle, that gout is exclusively an inflammatory affection of the ligamentous and tendinous structure; that it is merely
local *, and unknown as a constitutional complaint, but through the medium of morbid sympathies generated, and rendered more or less
inveterate by its protracted duration.

" The originality professed by me was that
of decidedly recommending the practice to public
adoption; not because it merely afforded alleviation to pain, but because such alleviation of pain
was justified by the nature of the disease, in
being a local and not a constitutional affection.
My claim to the refrigerant treatment of gouty
inflammation is not rested on so baseless a pre-
tence, as that of having been the first casually
to have subjected to trial the topical use of cold

but *that* of the principle on which its safety and salutary efficacy
are founded, is held, and maintained to be my peculiar, exclusive, and incontrovertible right.   K.

* We think this opinion will meet with general opposition,
Editors. Oppose it, *Editors*; neither the author nor his doctrine
will shrink from the contest.   K.

water:

water; but on the sure foundation of having justified, applied, and realized its indisputable efficacy, by a theory * which undauntedly aspires to be at once perfectly original, and *incontrovertibly* † rational.

"The opinion which has been hitherto held of gout, must have ever opposed an insuperable obstacle to a scientific adoption of reduced temperature for its cure, however glaring its incidental efficacy might have appeared, or however strongly recommended. The establishment of the remedy, therefore, was impossible, without the originality which is in my full (it may be presumed indisputable) right, that of considering gout as a *local* affection, wholly independent of constitutional origin.

"Neither my medical reading nor conversation had furnished the smallest clue to forming my opinion, which led me so far to neglect what had generally been written on gout, as to

---

* Fully given in a Dissertation, on the eve of being published by the author of this reply. See the preceding Dissertation on arthritis, or gout.   K.

† For incontrovertibly rational, the phrase in my manuscript, 'rational' only, is erroneously printed in the Medical and Physical Journal, No. 61, p. 243, l. 21.   K.

have

have overlooked all, and every of those *splendid authorities*, quoted by 'Constant Reader,' for the topical use of cold water in that disease *, Those quotations are totally useless, and quite irrelevant to the purpose for which they are adduced. They say no more than may be attested by the experience of many hundred individuals, that gouty pain may be subdued by the external application of cold water to the affected part, but with an avowed *dread* of the remedy being

---

* Since the publication of this reply, an interesting communication addressed to me, by an unprejudiced and experienced physician, whose name is not permitted at *present* to be publicly mentioned, contains, among other intelligent and valuable observations, the following appropriate remark on the unavailing result of searching medical records, whether ancient or modern, for any opinions on gouty affection, that tend either to elucidate its nature, or improve its treatment. Speaking of the want of salutary efficacy in the heating management of the disease, he adds, 'Being dissatisfied with a practice, however sanctioned, that was productive of so little advantage, I consulted every author from antiquity to Sydenham, and from Sydenham to Messrs. Cheyne, Grant, and Hill, without bettering either my practice or my own suffering.' This gentleman does me the honour to say, that my first publication on the refrigerant treatment of gout in the Medical and Physical Journal, confirmed his previous opinion of the validity of the principle on which the practice was therein founded, and determined him fully to adopt it in his own case. The issue he has promised to make known to me, which will probably not be lost to the public. K.

worse

worse than the disease. Hence the ground of
' Constant Reader's' triumphantly exclaiming,
It has been often tried, and as often abandoned.
Why has it been abandoned * ? ' Because its
safety had not the warranty of my doctrine for
its general, confident, and permanent adoption.
Plagiarism is my detestation, literary robbery
has a deep shade of moral turpitude; nor are the

---

* " Why has it been abandoned ?" After this phrase is inserted
in the Medical and Physical Journal, No. 61, p. 244, l. 4-5,
the sentence ' if it has ever really been abandoned.' My notes, my
recollection, and the consistency of my argument, concur to
authorize me in averring, that *this passage* was not in my manuscript sent for publication ; and that, therefore, it has been sur-
reptitiously foisted into the text (it matters not by whom) in
its passing from me to the public. The Editors are amenable
for all deviations from the original, and have here drawn on
themselves a serious responsibility, by most unjustifiably adding
what it must have been my object to avoid. The passage is particularly important : ' *If it has ever really been abandoned.*' No
doubt was entertained by me of its having been *necessarily* abandoned, whenever it might have been casually taken up, for
want of doctrinal justification. Why then should the Editors
esteem it convenient to make me say what could not have been
consistently said by me ? Was it to involve me in an absurd
inconsistency, or obliquely to dispute with me the sort of originality which was never claimed by me, that of having been the
first to have applied cold water to gouty inflammation ? This is
the counterpart of ' Constant Reader's ' conduct with the additional offence of making me the organ of my own opposition.
' *Nemo me impunè lacessit.*'   K.

epithets

epithets 'arrogant' and 'assuming' to be tolerated * from a 'shrouded' and vindictive assailant.

" If to claim a right which cannot be disproved is arrogance and assumption, then are these *gentle terms* applicable to the immortal Harvey and Jenner. Opponents were not wanting to dispute the discovery of the circulation of the blood with the former, nor have wranglers been remiss in endeavouring to garble the exclusive right of the latter to the establishment of vaccine inoculation. It was not sufficient to invalidate, or even disparage the exploring merit of Harvey, that others had preceded him in imagining that the blood flowed in a circular course; nor was the public value of vaccine inoculation at all diminished in favour of Jenner's originality, by others having previously,

---

* For ' *to be tolerated*,' the language of the original, the very *polite gentleness* of editorship has, with more than *poetic license*, substituted in No. 61, p. 244, l. 10, of the Medical and Physical Journal, ' *not to be deemed just or fair*.' Are the mild epithets *just* and *fair* applicable to an enraged anonymous writer, dealing in acrimonious invective, for having been discovered in endeavouring to palm on the public *falsehood* for *truth ?* But setting this aside, the objection is taken against the Editors of the Medical and Physical Journal, as faithful *reporters*, not *censors*, of subjects communicated to them for publication.   K.

but

but privately and incidentally inoculated. Such desultory procedure was useless, and must have ever remained so without doctrinal, systematic, and explanatory aid, to demonstrate its practical worth, and to ensure its public adoption.

" If, agreeably to ' Constant Reader's ' opinion of my want of originality in the refrigerant treatment of gout, the reputed efficacy of cold water, or reduced temperature, had remained on the authority of those who had recommended it, but who had not examined the nature of the disease sufficiently to perceive its perfect safety, and to entitle it to public acceptance, in what state would have been the practice at this moment? Would the gouty patient have immersed the affected limb in cold water oftener, or with more confidence, than the vaccine inoculation would have been substituted for the variolous, had the preventive efficacy of the former remained unpromulgated, and unestablished by its able advocate? It may be objected, the parallel does not hold. As it respects comparative originality it does most perfectly. As it regards utility, time only can determine the question; but the probationary period which has already elapsed, since the commencement of my investi-

5

gation

gation of the subject, promises fully to establish the parallel also in point of utility.

" If immediate relief, without the slightest inconvenience to the general health, ascribable to early cure, can entitle reduced temperature to be considered as an infallibly efficacious remedy for gout, hundreds can already attest its irresistible claim to that character; and, in spite of ' shrouded,' or unshrouded opposition, its salutary influence will be progressively gaining increasing confidence, and soon prove the nature and degree of my right to originality, in scientifically authorizing and establishing the topical use of reduced heat in gouty inflammation.

" I now take my leave in turn of your ' shrouded' correspondent, without the smallest dread of his unshrouded ' goose-quill *' endeavour to ' throw cold water' on my book when it shall appear. Indeed, this wondrous witty, this 'goose-quill' threat, savours too much of goose cackle to be at all terrific.

' Vox, et præterea nihil.'

* Erroneously printed ' goose quills' in the Medical and Physical Journal, No. 61, p. 245, l. 15. K.

" Saying

" Saying no more of what is past, it may not
be deemed uncharitable at parting, to desire
' Constant Reader ' to be extremely cautious in
again dabbling in *misrepresentation*, and, what is
worse, in being displeased at detection. If, after
this warning, he should be again caught tripping
over the sacred boundary of truth, and that in
his '*propria persona*' majesty, he must expect
no quarter from me; he will be deservedly consigned to literary infamy, and be for ever proscribed all claim to credit.

" Until, however, this said ' Constant Reader '
shall think proper to quit his lurking-hole, and
appear in his threatened ' *propria persona*,' he
will be too despicable a combatant for my encounter. When he shall actually skulk from
his snarling retreat he will start as fair game,
and it is possible that the *undisguised* friends of
medical improvement in general, and more particularly the numerous votaries to my gouty
remedy, will join me in a *hue* and *cry* against
this *mighty unshrouding champion*, and laugh to
scorn his impotent * but malignant design of
' *throwing cold water* ' on a scientific and humane
endeavour to establish the infallible efficacy

* *Impotent* in the original, erroneously printed ' impatient '
in the Medical and Physical Journal, No. 61, p. 245, l. 38. K.

of

of that fluid, in promptly and safely curing gouty inflammation.

' Spectatum admissi, risum teneatis amici.'

" Conscious of the rectitude of my intention, and of my indefeasible claim to that originality, which confers a right to discovery, and which alone is worth contending for; also fully persuaded of the important advantages already rendered to mankind by my doctrine and practice in gouty affection; my publication on the subject will be ushered into the world without any solicitude as to its fate. Whatever may be its defects, its intrinsic merits promise long, *very long*, to survive the hostile machinations, the daring but pitiful efforts of prejudice, calumny, malevolence, misrepresentation, and all the other ignoble passions, whether ' *shrouded* ' or *unshrouded*, oral, or ' *goose-quilled*,' bilious,' or ' *jocular*.'

' Rusticus expectat dum defluat amnis
' Labitur, et labetur in omne volubilis ævum.'

" I am, &c.

" *Taunton,*
February 5, 1804. " ROBERT KINGLAKE."

x *Cases*

*Cases of rheumatic and arthritic Inflammation suc-
cessfully treated by the topical Use of diminished
Temperature; by Mr. Taylor, Surgeon.—Extracted from the Medical and Physical Journal
for the Month of April 1804.*

"To the Editors of the Medical and Physical
Journal.

"Gentlemen,

"The subject of gout having been lately
brought forward in the Medical and Physical
Journal, in consequence of the treatment proposed for its cure by Dr. Kinglake, I shall
make no apology for troubling you with the following observations. It is not my intention to
enter into the controversy that has taken place
between Dr. Kinglake and 'a Constant Reader,'
but merely to state facts as they have come to
my knowledge. The application of cold water,
with a view of reducing morbid excess of temperature, does not appear to be a new remedy, but
on the contrary; and, like many other remedies for disease, has been laid aside, and after a
time resumed *.

"I have

* It has not been held to be a new remedy, but contended
that its use in *gouty inflammation* has been hitherto incidental,
desultory, fearful, and wholly unauthorized by any consistent
view

" I have always been in the habit, since I began medical practice, of using cold water as a topical application in local inflammations of the joints; but since Dr. Kinglake's communications, I have employed it in every case of acute rheumatism, as well as gout, which has fallen under my care, and am happy to say with uniform success, in cutting short the disease *. Many instances could be produced by me to prove, that the application of cold water is not only a perfectly safe remedy in gout and rheumatism, but a highly beneficial one. The following is a case of acute rheumatism, in which it was used with decided advantage.

" J. Stockdale, aged twenty-three years, was attacked in January last with severe febrile symptoms, pain and swelling in the ankles, knees, and wrists; the pain was very violent, particularly at night, and when in bed. He had been ill

view of the nature of the disease. For want of this advantage, the practice never has, and without it never could be generally, confidently, and permanently adopted.   K.

* This candid acknowledgment of the ingenious author, liberally disclaims having been led to the practice by any analogical view of gouty and other inflammations, such as has been affirmed to have been the original ground of my subjecting it to trial, and on ascertaining its salutary efficacy, of recommending it to public adoption.   K.

a week

a week when I saw him, and had been attacked
on the day previous to my visit with a violent
fixed pain under the left breast, extending to
the clavicle, attended with a cough and difficulty
of breathing; he expectorated a considerable
quantity of bloody mucus. He was ordered to
take ten drops of the tinctura digitalis, every
four hours, in a glass of cold water, and fifteen
grains of pulv. ipecac. comp. at night at bed-
time; the joints were directed to be kept constantly wet with cloths, dipped in a lotion, composed of water, coloured with tinctura lavendulæ
composita. On visiting him the next day, I
found he had rested better, was freer from pain,
and the swelling somewhat diminished; but as
his breathing was still impeded, and cough
troublesome, it was deemed proper to apply a
blister to the side. The tinct. digitalis, and
pulv. ipecac. comp. were continued as before,
and the red lotion applied to the tumefied parts,
which he was eagerly desirous of having renewed
every few minutes, as it made him so comfortable
and easy. He went on mending rapidly, and,
in the course of seven or eight days from my first
seeing him, the swelling and pain had subsided,
his fever and cough had left him, and he had
not a symptom of disease but general debility,
for which he took half a dram of bark three
times

times a day. It is to be remarked that this patient had been seized with this disease about six weeks before, in a slight degree, from which he soon recovered, but having imprudently exposed himself to wet, brought on this second attack.

" From a variety of cases, in which cold water has, by my direction, been applied to arthritic inflammation, I shall deem it necessary to state only one, as they would all tend to establish the same point, viz. the efficacy and propriety of the remedy. Mrs. B. between fifty and sixty years of age, has been subject to the attack of gout, in one or both feet, for several years. She has usually had two or three fits in the year, and those generally tedious and very painful ones. In last December she was attacked with inflammation and swelling in both feet ; the pain was very severe. I saw her the day after the coming on of the fit, and proposed the application of the red lotion ; but, as Mrs. B. had always been in the habit of applying warmth, by flannel, &c. she for some time objected to the application of cold, and it was no easy matter for me to overcome her prejudices ; however, she consented, and cloths well wetted were wrapped round the feet, and kept constantly

upon

upon them; the almost immediate effects of which were, an abatement of the pain; and, by continuing the application, she was in three days completely cured of the complaint, a little stiffness and debility of the feet only remaining for a few days more.

" The patient was, as may be readily conceived, highly pleased with the remedy, and not a little surprised at its beneficial influence in so short a period *.

" I am, &c.

" THOMAS TAYLOR, Surgeon."

" Harleston, Norfolk,
March 6th, 1804.

---

* It would be even illiberal to suppose it possible for incredulity, however warped by prejudice, to resist the assurances here given of the salutary efficacy of reduced temperature in arthritic or rheumatic affection, were it not that inconceivable instances are still occurring of unyielding opposition to similar facts, enforced by an equal degree of demonstrative proof. The popular cry is, Oh, it must be hurtful, it is so contrary to the prevailing opinion of what is useful. This may be excused as the unmeaning exclamation of prejudice; but science must lament that medical practitioners are yet to be found, who, without having known a single example of its having proved injurious, endeavour to terrify and dissuade the public from the practice, by insinuating that, though it temporarily relieves pain, it will sooner or later destroy life. Is not this grossly violating the established rules of correct argumentation? is it not the *petitio principii*

Observations and Case of " Perscrutator," in Reply to " Medicus."—Extracted from the Medical and Physical Journal, for the Month of June 1804.

" To the Editors of the Medical and Physical Journal.

" Gentlemen,

" Any thing like vindictive controversy, or replication of illiberality or malevolence, ought

principii of logical subterfuge, the *begging of the question,* which facts cannot support? It is indeed a subject of just and proud exultation for the liberal advocates of the refrigerant treatment of gouty disease, that amidst all the opposition and disgraceful animosity with which the investigation has been assailed, but *one fact* has yet been publicly adduced to discredit the practice, and that *solitary fact* was the case of the late Dr. Gregory, published by an anonymous author, calling himself a " Constant Reader;" which pretended fact has since been publicly proved and acknowledged to be false, and does strongly appear to have been a malicious fabrication. Doubtful points can only be elucidated by the clear evidence of facts; on this testimony the cooling treatment of gout is broadly and securely founded; it asks no other support, its importance rests its remedial value exclusively on it; and yet, instances, which should compel belief, are still often disparaged, misrepresented, and deemed inadmissible: disbelief, thus circumstanced, is grounded on nothing rationally questionable, but on either a thoughtless or inveterate determination to withhold assent. To such senseless and obstinate refusal no successful appeal can be made, nor indeed would its acquiescence confer any authority. K.

to be universally deprecated and scouted; but in
what manner such have (as Medicus * has asserted in your last Journal) tended more to
embarrass than to elucidate the science of medicine, demands a more satisfactory proof than
mere suggestion.   What has excited controversy
of such obnoxious contexture, seems to be the

---

* This *self-named* " *Medicus*" discovers in his observations
(published in the Medical and Physical Journal for April 1804,
pages 348, 349, 350, 351), the peevish captiousness, and
deficient talent, so conspicuous in the memorable strictures of
" *Constant Reader*." Has his *constant reading* of the Medical and
Physical Journal advanced him to the rank of " *Medicus ?*" or,
without having any title to that appellation, has he availed himself of it to " *shroud*" his notoriety as " *Constant Reader ?*"   If
this suspicion be unfounded, the force of the resemblance justifies its being entertained.   Should, however, two distinct
authors have been actually concerned in these productions, it
must be allowed that the strictest unison obtains between them,
in coarseness of diction, total want of authority, and contradic-
tory mode of arguing.   Nor does the critical and approving
discernment of the Editors of the Medical and Physical Journal,
implied by admitting such futile remarks, appear advantageously
contrasted.   Indeed, the glaring, the unworthy partiality shewn
by those Editors to every objection publicly made to my doctrine and treatment of gout, and the unwarrantable manner in
which they have thought proper to mutilate and misrepresent
my last reply, authorize me in saying, that if they themselves
have not actually indulged their opposition under the fictitious
names of " *Constant Reader*" and " *Medicus*," they have, by
their uneditorlike conduct, invited and patronised the several
anonymous attacks against me, published in their Journal.   K.

fair

fair relation and detail of certain experiments, or the result of individual practice, upon the salutary operation of cold affusion in arthritic paroxysms. From the recent introduction of this mode of treatment of gout, has arisen a conflict, which, although it has little or no claim to candour, nor is it indicative of benevolent interest for public welfare, is certainly incapable of degrading your Journal *, embarrassing the science, or sinking the exalted establishment of medical inquiry into contumelious puerility.

" I must conclude with 'Medicus,' that theories are very often intended more to convey plausible and ingenious opinions of subtle speculatists, than to lead to a prompt and successful practice; yet I cannot but observe, that whatever may be our deficiencies in our knowledge of the operations of the nervous system, there may be good room for cautious experiments, and warrantable deviations from general practice,

* The Journal alluded to has surely not been degraded by having been the vehicle of information of incalculable importance to the healing art; but it has been most sorrily so in stooping, in the first instance, to report a *very improbable* narrative as a fact, from an *anonymous author*; and after that pretended fact had been *publicly refuted*, in lending itself to the base revenge of detected falsehood.   K.

if

if they are derived from strict analogy, and supported by a successful issue.

" It much surprises me, that ' Medicus,' who starts as a reformer of medical discussion, and the strong advocate for the plain and simple detail of all means, from the weakest to the most potent, conducive to the cure of disease, should so far forget himself, as not only to fall into the defects, of which he so much complains in others, but also, that he should depreciate the merits and the good effects derived from the practice of cold ablution in gouty affection. According to him, the *practise is contrary to all sound experience* * ; not *one instance* †, however, does he record where he observed its pernicious effects. Instead of facts, he contents himself with assertions.

* This sound experience, by some *heterogeneous* transformation, conceivable only to such mysterious *sages* as " Medicus," results from unsound prejudice. To common apprehension, indeed, it is no experience at all; it is no more than the puling hantling of Ignorance, generated by Cabal and fostered by Malevolence.　　　　　　　　　　　　　　K.

† In fact, not *one instance* exists, though, it is true, " Constant Reader" fabricated one; but, unhappily for the views of misrepresentation, it was too decidedly falsified to admit of a hope that an early attempt in the same way would prove more successful.

　　　　　　　　　　　　　　　　　K.

" If

" If gout be a general disease (as ' Medicus' believes it to be), why should not local means contribute to the cure, or remove that local affection which is the principal part of the disease; the removal of which, as in many cases of symptomatic affections, might accelerate the progress of a general, or at least temporary cure of the whole? But we know as little concerning the causes of diseases in general, especially of gout, or how they induce diseases, as we do of nervous operations; and in how many instances do we endeavour to cure general morbid action by destroying the principal leading symptoms? But the grand question seems to be, whether the gout be a local or general affection; or whether, after the frequent repetitions of its severity, it may not become catinated with, or form general morbid sympathies * ? Now should the gout be originally a general disease, there can be no pathological reason why the practice of local means,

* Although the local origin of gout is often obscured by habitual, accidental, and sympathetic affections of the system, yet it is always sufficiently distinct to evince, that its protraction on the affected part will exasperate any general disease which may have previously existed, and associatively generate new ailment in the exact ratio of the degree of local pain and the length of its continuance. Hence the strong, the cogent warranty for its speedy relief.   K.

which

which vanquishes the most harassing symptom, should not induce a salutary change in the diseased movement of the animal machine, and, by that process, produce a restoration of its healthy faculties. By the same rule, these diseased sympathies, arising from local arthritic affections, should gout be primarily unconnected with the system, may be interrupted ; and more salutary, or the accustomed healthy action redintegrated by the mere influence of local remedies.

" Let the opinion of medical men rest upon either side of the question, no ground can be tenable for uncandid and inefficient declamation; and a stubborn inflexibility in opposing practical and laudable innovation is more injurious to science than the greatest absurdity of the most flimsy hypothesis *.

" I could

---

* It must be impartially confessed, the criticism of " Medicus" is here ably controverted by " Perscrutator." The talents and liberality of the latter indeed, whoever he may be, had no difficult task to accomplish; but he has executed it with much appropriate judgment. Idle declamation vanishes before adverse facts, nor can canting pretensions to correctness, candour, and modesty be ever admitted as *real*, by the honest and discriminating. " Perscrutator" has generously volunteered his superior opposition to the wanton, the puerile hostility of " Medicus," against a practice which he audaciously says is *contrary to all sound* *exherience*,

* I could adduce as many instances in support
of the efficacy of the reduction of temperature
in gouty paroxysms, by cold water, as 'Medicus' has supposed instances contraindicative of
its use or inadmissibility; but I shall content myself in the relation of a single instance, where
the application of cold water was attended with
the happiest result. In this case it was not
directed by practical experience or legitimate
speculation, but by the mere instinctive impulse
of the suffering victim *.

experience, though he does not, *he can not*, adduce *a single instance* in support of his assertion, whilst he is confronted with
many in which it has proved most salutary. "Perscrutator"
is entitled to my best acknowledgment for refuting malevolence,
and exhibiting folly, in a manner worthy of his enlightened and
independent mode of reasoning. The attack savoured too
much of the "*shrouded*" malignancy of "Constant Reader," to
merit any *consideration* from me, much less a reply. K.

* It has been incidentally observed in the preceding dissertation, that the sense of feeling is an unerring guide in inflammatory pain to the appropriate remedy. Natural impulse re-
cognises its legitimacy, and would be invariably directed by it,
but for the marring counsels of perverted science, which by
arrogantly endeavouring to new-model, grossly misinterpret,
and but too often fatally disorder the vital ordinances of the
animal economy. The heating treatment of gout is a lamentable
example of the disastrous influence of scientific delusion in repugnance to every law of sensual temperature. K.

"A super-

" A superintendant of a fishery in Newfoundland, labouring under a gouty paroxysm, and, as is usual, strongly advised to remain confined in his room, suffered severely from the pain and great inflammation in one of his feet; but wishing to discharge his official duties, he became determined, against all persuasion, to go to sea in one of the fishing vessels. He silenced all opposition to his resolve, by crying out that his pain and the heat of the affected part were so great, he was confident nothing could abate them but cold; and if that did not relieve him, he would as soon die at sea as suffer so much torment in bed. The consequence was, that the poor sufferer was carried to the vessel, in which he put to sea, and was obliged, as is usual, to remain for several hours nearly up to his knees in salt water. In this situation, to the great astonishment of every one present, the pain and inflammation abated, and the man ceased to complain; on his return home, he insisted on his wet clothes remaining upon him, and in case of the symptoms returning, to have buckets of sea-water in readiness. By this treatment he always procured relief, and his habits of living induced many severe accessions almost every year, for which he would be carried into the sea, and there remain until the accustomed alleviation

. alleviation of his symptoms took place ; besides this, he had the inflamed parts wrapped in cloths immersed in the same fluid, which never failed of procuring the desired relief *.

" PERSCRUTATOR."

" *St. George's Place, Blackfriars Road,*
    April 10th, 1804.

---

* This very remarkable instance of the beneficial effects of topical refrigeration in gouty disease strikingly resembles the case of the fisherman, hereafter detailed by Mr. Montagu. The analogy indeed is so close as to lessen the objection which might be otherwise taken against it, from its wanting a real signature. It is not my wish to raise anonymous cases to the character of medical evidence; they are clearly not entitled to it; but they may, without trenching on the safety of truth, be admitted as corroborative testimony, particularly when recommended by every appearance of probability. Under the name of "*Constant Reader*" the world has been told that the late Dr. Gregory was suddenly killed by bathing his feet in cold water, when in a state of gouty inflammation. The event was too improbable, *inconceivable* indeed; it was questioned, refuted, and exposed. Under the name of " Perscrutator" the public is informed of a singularly inveterate case of gout having been speedily relieved and cured by topical cold, without any subsequent injury to the general health. The event is highly probable, is at issue with any attempt to falsify it; nay, kindred instances of salutary efficacy rest the fact on an immutable law of nature, and challenge its visionary adversaries to *authenticate* a single instance in which topical cold has proved injurious in gouty inflammation. K.

Case

Case and Observations communicated by Dr. Clarke.

" *To Dr. Kinglake.*

" Dear Sir,

" Having received much satisfaction from reading your observations and treatment of gout, and gouty affections, in the Medical Journal, permit me the liberty of addressing you, not only to assent to your opinions, but to add an instance of the efficacy of cold applications over hot ones; and the impropriety, not to say worse, of applying flannel and other heating substances to a part already in a state of inflammation.

" Upon the first attack of gout, rheumatism, or rheumatic gout (for I have experienced the three pretty distinctly *), many years ago, I heated

---

* The ingenious author here, conformably to established prejudice, adopts the prevailing distinctions assigned to the different degrees of gouty inflammation occurring in different temperamental and accidental states for morbid impression. If the various modes under which different degrees of the same disease may appear, deserve to be distinguished by appropriate names, the several titles of gout, rheumatism, and rheumatic gout, may, from the familiarity which they have respectively acquired, be practically retained; but when the question of such nominal propriety is extended to scientific authority, it is contended, that

it

treated the disorder in myself, as well as others, in the usual mode, and I believe exactly with the same success; that of sometimes alleviating, but neither shortening nor expelling the complaint. Being dissatisfied with a practice, however sanctioned, that was productive of so little advantage, I consulted every author from antiquity to Sydenham, and from Sydenham to Messrs. Cheyne, Grant, and Hill, without bettering either my practice or my own sufferings *. I have at different times made use of a great variety of external applications, and once ventured to blister the pained part ; an experiment that by no means, from my own feelings, would I recommend others to try ; but every applica-

It may be decidedly resisted on the philosophical ground of there being no radical difference in these variously denominated forms of disease : in all of them, the ligamentous and tendinous structure is held to be the genuine seat of the affection, however diversified its external character. K.

* It will have been seen that this passage has been quoted in a former note in this Appendix, with a remark of my not being at liberty to mention the author's name. It was desired at that time, that the above communication should not be published, until the effects of the cooling treatment of gout had been more fully ascertained in the author's own case. Since then the restriction has been removed, by the author having acquired the additional knowledge he wanted, as will appear in the sequel of his transmitted intelligence. K.

tion,

tion, of the stimulant or sedative kind, made use of, failed in producing any good effect. I therefore submitted to patience and flannel, till I found, that by the different attacks I had to fear the loss of the use of my limbs, from direct debility, induced by one attack supervening another, before the limbs had recovered their lost tone. In this state I had, previous to your communication of the effects of cold water, determined upon trying the shower-bath, and had actually constructed one upon a larger scale than usual, and only waited a change of weather to put my plan in execution, when your paper upon the subject made its appearance, and confirmed me in my design, which I put in practice, and continued through last summer, and did intend pursuing through the winter, but a severe cold obliged me to desist *.

"In November last I was seized as usual with an attack in the ankle, which had every appearance of confining me for a month or six

* The intelligent author (as acknowledged in a subsequent letter) was not led to the use of cold water by any opinion of its efficacy in reducing the morbid excess of heat common to gouty and every other kind of inflammatory disease, but from its reputed tonic virtue, with a view to strengthen the enfeebled limbs, and to obviate eventual decrepitude.   K.

weeks.

weeks. I immediately had recourse to cold ablution, which eased the pain, abated the swelling, and allowed me the next day to walk and
to be upon my feet in the wet and cold three
hours. When I got home, I immediately had recourse to the cold water again, which I repeated
every evening till the pain and swelling were
gone (about a week). About three weeks ago I
had a fresh attack (after exposure in the cold and
moisture) in the ankle, more severe than the
former one, and exactly similar to those attacks
from which I suffered much pain and long confinement. I had immediate recourse to cold
ablution, with the same effect, abatement of
pain and swelling, and, after two days confinement, was again able to attend my professional
calls, and walk with tolerable ease.

" Upon Friday last a fresh attack seized the
left knee, attended with pain, debility, great
soreness upon the slightest touch, and some
degree of redness and swelling. As this put on a
serious appearance, I was obliged to apply the
cold water three or four times a day *. Upon

* It should have been applied at least as often, during *every
hour*, to have early and duly extinguished the inflammatory
heat, and to have prevented sympathetic excitement on other
joints. K.

Y 2 Sunday

Sunday I was enabled to go out as usual, though
I still feel great weakness at this moment of
writing, and have every reason to expect a fresh
assault upon the right knee.

" It is necessary to premise, that the general
course the disorder used to pursue, was an attack
upon the toe, metatarsal bones, or heel of one
foot; after a torture of some days to shift to the
opposite knee, from thence to the opposite
foot, and thence to the knee of the same side.
May not the different attacks I have experienced
in each foot, and now in each knee, shew the
disposition of the disease to have gone its usual
round, but that its progress has been arrested by
cold applications * ?

" Allow me to ask one question, should you
think the above worth the honour of an answer,
Does your experience authorize me to continue

* The morbid disposition to gouty disease has been indeed
strongly marked and actively developed in the successive attacks
which occurred. The progress of the affection, it is true, has
been repressed, but much more would probably have been
effected by a more assiduous use of topical cold. With such
aid, the disease would have been most likely confined to a state
of dormant disposition only, in the joints which were subse-
quently and sympathetically affected, and not have proceeded to
inflammatory excitement.   K.

                                                        my

my attack of the disease from joint to joint, should it repeatedly occur * ?

" Should you think it deserving attention, my mode of treating myself will be at your service, and I will most cordially thank you for any hint or improvement which may have occurred to you in practice. I shall pursue the cold plan to its utmost extent, not only to put off a present attack, but, by its use, endeavour to prevent a future one †.

* My answer to this question was given decidedly in the affirmative. My experience had fully warranted me in pursuing with topical cold every shifting of gouty excitement, and repeated instances had farther taught me, that, promptly and effectually to subdue the fleeting transpositions of gouty ailment, every joint which may have been either originally or sympathetically the seat of the disease, or whether suffering alternately or synchronously, should be unremittedly kept in the temperature of cold water, until every remnant of painful heat be allayed. By this procedure, every source of recurrent irritation, whether original or sympathetic, will be completely annihilated. K.

† The author, with a correctness of investigation worthy of science, and with a warmth of benevolence honourable to his feelings, has subjected his own case of gouty disease to a scrutinizing trial of the effects of reduced temperature. His report has hitherto been highly favourable to the remedy: the prosecution of his laudable inquiry, detailed in the subsequent letter, will be found to be not less impartial than instructive. K.

" About

" About fifteen years ago the disorder began its attack, at the age of thirty-three, and very year since has not allowed me many months ease.

" I am,

" Dear Sir,

" With respect, &c.

" C. M. CLARKE."

" *Louth,*
February 21*st,* 1804.

Second Communication by Dr. Clarke, on the Treatment of gouty Affection.

" *To Dr. Kinglake.*

" Dear Sir,

" Your letter, of the 6th of March last, I had the satisfaction of receiving, and repent much that I should have so wrongly directed my former one to you. Believe me, Sir, I should long ago have done myself the honour of answering your very polite, satisfactory, and friendly letter, but I had, as I conceived, strong reasons from time to time to postpone that pleasure, as I wished to give you the most minute detail respecting myself, and the conduct I pursued, so far as may benefit others, or give you that information which may, in your hands, be extended to others ; being a proper subject to
make

make a trial upon, having had, as I before informed you, so many attacks of gout, or rheumatic gout, that a serious debility was evidently
seizing me from head to foot, accompanied with
dyspepsia and its train of uneasy sensations, and
internal weakness. Frequent confinement, and
lying for weeks upon my back, had also brought
on an affection of the kidnies, which still in
some measure remains; but at one time the relaxation was so great as to affect the neck of the
bladder. If I retained the urine a little beyond
the time that the inclination for passing it first
began, I could not restrain the flow, until no
more remained to be evacuated, and even then
had not for some time any power over the
sphincter muscle.*. In my habit of visiting
gouty patients, some of them men of the world
and fortune, I evidently saw that the old *regime*
was not to be entirely trusted to. Like them, I
was (if possible) determined not to be, nor de-

* The systematic debility, which results from frequent relapses, and the protracted duration of gouty disease, is in general
preponderately felt in the alimentary canal and urinary passages,
and shewn in the relative symptoms of indigestion, oppression,
flatulence, intestinal griping, constipation, renal pain, and irregular secretion and excretion of urine. The long continuance
of the recumbent posture also much contributes to these morbid effects, both by partial pressure, and want of locomotive
exertion.   K.

prived

prived of the use of my limbs, as many of them were. Every means I adopted to put off and keep off the attacks. Steam (which I see mentioned lately) years ago I tried. I had a tin kettle with different tubes, so formed as to be lengthened or shortened at pleasure, that the steam might be conveyed from the kettle upon the fire to a settee, chair, &c. and applied to the limb affected; but I found as little relief as from blistering, leeches, and other external applications of every kind *. Almost in despair, I looked forward to the application of cold as my only resource. Until I read your paper in the Medical Journal, I candidly confess, I only considered cold as a simple

* The steam of either water, or any other fluid, is in no intelligible view of its efficacy adapted directly to remedy a disease (like that of gout) of excessive temperature. To be active, it must be the vehicle of a degree of heat that would inordinately stimulate and exhaust motive power, and thus indirectly induce a state of debility on the inflamed parts, incompatible with inflammatory action. In that case pain might be alleviated, but the burning severity to which the diseased parts would have been subjected, would necessarily leave them in a state of extreme weakness, perhaps even of damaged structure, and certainly with an increased susceptibility for morbid impression. When aqueous steam distributes to surrounding *media* its vaporific temperature, it condenses into tepid water, and is then neither stimulant enough to exasperate gouty inflammation, nor sufficiently refrigerant to reduce its excessive heat. It is therefore either noxiously excitant or quite inert.   K.

tonic,

tonic, and hoped by its use to recover the tone of the system, that I might be better enabled to undergo any future attacks. I did not at that time consider its utility in either preventing or removing the complaint when actually present: for that information and hint I find myself indebted to you *.

*"Since receiving your last letter, I have not been sparing in the use of cold ablution, indeed I do it every night. I have experienced, after a little necessary fatigue, so much pain and restlessness, that my feet were uneasy in either a standing, sitting, or an horizontal position. I could rest in no place or posture long; all this I have as constantly removed, by ordering a basin of cold pump water, and having my feet washed, with cloths wetted and put upon them, holding my feet over the basin, and renewing the soaked cloths whenever the water was drained from them; after this, I have passed the evening without pain, or any uneasy feeling. If I am cold, I still apply the water in the evening. If I have took cold I do not desist; if the pain

* This liberal acknowledgment evinces the ingenuousness and love of truth with which the author has been actuated in his speculations on gouty disease. K.

attacks

attacks my knees, I persevere, and am at this moment infinitely better than I have been for years *.

" I have experienced as yet no attack to confine me, and have every reason, from my feelings, from my state of health, from an increase of strength, and from being able to make more exertions than usual, to persevere and carry on the present plan to its utmost extent. I propose immediately beginning with the cold bath, and going on with it †.

---

* Hence it appears that a distempered state of motive excitability, shewn in the low or aching degree only of diseased sensation, may be checked and prevented from proceeding to the aggravated stage of inflammatory violence, by the sedulous use of topical cold. This fact proves the propriety of attempting, by reduced temperature, to counteract both the primary accession and relapse of gouty attacks, when the approach of either may be indicated by uneasy feeling in any of the joints. This uneasiness is more particularly liable to occur towards the close of the day, from the stimulant influence of the natural evening paroxysm of fever. Cold water, topically applied to the painful joints in the evening, is therefore peculiarly seasonable, and likely to be more beneficial than at any other time.　　K.

† General cold bathing promises, in the existing circumstances, by duly restoring systematic energy, strengthening the enfeebled joints, and establishing a salutary distribution of temperature, to protect the constitutional excitability at large, and more particularly that of the ligamentous and tendinous structure, from either transiently painful, or inflammatory disorder.　　　　　　　　　　　　　　K.

" Should

" Should any new idea have struck you, or
any extension of the mode of the application of
cold, do me the favour of letting me know, and
I will give it a trial; so thoroughly am I convinced, that, to obtain a temporary alleviation
of pain, a lasting injury has been done to the
constitution, by the application of heat. It has
increased the relaxation so much, as nearly to
have destroyed the energy of the circulation in
the extremities, and decrepitude has been the
consequence *. In not hastily answering your
letter, I hope the satisfaction I feel in expressing
my present situation will plead as an apology.
I need not say how very happy I should be,
whenever a vacant hour should occur, in hearing
from you †.

" I am,

" Dear Sir,

" *Louth*,   " With great respect,
June 3d, 1804.   " C. M. CLARKE."

Cases

* This relaxation and failure of vascular energy in the extremities arise from the indirect debility induced by the noxious excitement of excessive temperature, exasperated and protracted by
heating treatment.   K.

† The author of this communication has, by the extent and
persevering zeal of his researches into the efficacy of topical cold
in gouty disease, richly merited the exalted distinction of being
a public benefactor to mankind. It is to such humane endea-

vours

Cases communicated by Mr. Montagu.

" To Dr. Kinglake.

" Sir,

" Finding, by your letter of January last, that it is your intention to publish, for the general benefit, your experiments on topical application of cold in arthritic inflammation ; it would, in my opinion, be important, that facts collected from as many quarters as possible, unconnected with your professional treatment, should be brought in view, in order to keep down the stubborn prejudices of mankind, which at all times militate so much against the enlargement of science, and the expansion of the intellectual faculties.

" With this view, I take the liberty of informing you, that since my last letter to you, stating

vours to ascertain the real virtue of proposed remedies, that the practice of medicine owes its most valuable improvements. To similar exertions are due the cooling treatment of the small-pox, and the hopeful prospect of the management of fever being hereafter implicitly directed by the indications of sensual temperature. A wanton attempt at innovation in the cure of diseases, is worse than trifling, is dangerously frivolous; but to plead the privilege of custom, as an unassailable sanctuary; for unfounded and hurtful prejudice, is to prefer error to correctness, and injury to benefit.   K.

my

my own ease, I have tried the use of cold water on a servant, who it seems has a gouty habit, though a gardener, and consequently inured to hard labour *. But it is proper first to inform you, he is a free liver, and, to shew the difference in the effects of gout, when treated in the two opposite extremes, that he was about the same time last year seized with the gout in his hands and feet, extending to his knees, and by living generously, as is usually recommended; and having no objection to such a regimen, he took two pints of gin per diem, viz. within the twenty-four hours, besides a large portion of white-ale (an inebriating liquor peculiar to Devonshire, drank in a state of fermentation). By this plan he was confined to his bed three months, in continual gout and excruciating torture, was a

---

* Hard labour, by assisting the digestion of food, by appropriately distributing alimentary sustenance over the system, and by obviating morbid plenitude, diminishes the number of remote causes of arthritic affection ; but by subjecting the ligamentous and tendinous structure to violent exertions, it tends to disorder its salutary temperature, to unduly stretch its constituent fibres, and to induce that painful inflammatory disease termed sprain, which, in the preceding Dissertation, has been identified with the essential nature of gouty ailment. Hence, though the labourer is not exposed to the action of the more common remote causes of gout, yet he is not exempted from that of variable temperature, and excessive motion of the joints. K.

cripple

cripple for a long time, and in fact will never have so complete use of his limbs as before.

" On this inflammatory subject, so full of phlogiston, who was again attacked this spring, I thought a fair opportunity offered of trying the vast power cold water seems to have, particularly in arthritic inflammation. I found him in my garden with one hand wrapped in flannel, and prodigiously swollen, the pain of which had kept him awake all night. I made him instantly take off all the covering, and plunge his hand repeatedly in a tub of cold water, which happened to be near, and I ordered him to do the same frequently during the day, and at night, and the next morning, to use wet cloths, as you recommend. By this seasonable application, and a prohibition of spirits, though I allowed him a quart of white-ale per day, his hand soon got well.

" In three days after his first seizure, a violent paroxysm attacked his feet and ankles, attended with great inflammation on these parts; the same application was made very frequently with equal success, without any return to his hand; but it was followed by a violent paroxysm on both knees.

5

knees. At this time his courage nearly failed him, partly perhaps by the influence of the illiterate, who most likely told him it would kill him; and though he was convinced that the cold water had restored his hand and feet, and at all times gave instant relief, yet persuaded by his equals about him, he thought it drove it only from one part to another, forgetting the state of combustion his blood was in, from his general mode of life. However, after suffering much pain for some time, and weakened for want of rest and the usual support of drams, cold water was again applied, and the consequence was, that in five days after he was at work in my garden, and walked without a stick. A slight paroxysm again took possession of one knee; but the same remedy, and two or three days rest from labour, without confinement, also restored that limb; and he is now, about three weeks from his first attack, stronger on his feet than he was in five months after his former fit, treated with heat externally and internally, and is now mowing my walks.

" You will see I have not entered minutely into detail, but have related the substance of a case, than which there cannot be a greater proof

of

of the powerful efficacy of cold application, continued with perseverance *.

"I shall

* This case, as its intelligent communicator justly observes,
clearly evinces the vast power of cold water in reducing
arthritic inflammation, and how beneficial its unremitted application ultimately proves in the most unpromising circumstances
of the disease. Neither the broken strength nor vitiated excitability, induced by habitual intemperance, could resist the
salutary efficacy of topical cold in gouty irritation. Nor did its
sympathetic transference to the other joints in any shape involve
the general health in disease. Nor can it ever do so. The
morbid action is associatively excited on kindred structure only.
It cannot by any law of physical sympathy strictly occur on any
vital part. The visceral organs are not constituted of the dense
texture of ligaments and tendons, and are therefore neither
originally nor sympathetically susceptible of gouty inflammation,
which exclusively appertains to that fabric. Gouty disease may
indeed impair the general health, and even destroy life, by its
unmitigated and prolonged pain; incessant irritation from an
unhealing and ill-conditioned sore may do the same; but in both
cases the systematic injury flows *solely* from a local source, and
may be obviated by a seasonable removal of the cause. The
torture of the ligamentous and tendinous inflammation, or gout,
may sympathetically pervade and actuate the whole frame, distemper the general heat, agitate the arterial system, derange the
due distribution of the circulating fluids, induce headach, delirium, difficult respiration, sickness, vomiting, thirst, hot and
dry skin, &c. But are not all these *common symptoms* of general
irritation arising from *local pain?* Do they not prove the nature
and magnitude of the evil from whence they proceed, and furnish the strongest argument for the urgent necessity of its cure?
Early remedy, in the very teeth of opposing prejudice, is alone
calculated

" I shall now close this by informing you, there is a fisherman in this neighbourhood, who is a martyr to the gout, who assures me that, as soon he as can crawl upon his hands and feet from his house to the beach, which is very near, he always plunges into the sea, and suffers the water to flow over him, and that, without assigning any cause, he finds instant relief and daily restoration of health, and strength of limbs, though, from living almost entirely upon gin, and without much solids, he has long been incapable of holding an oar in his hand, being so distorted.

calculated to prevent the morbid sympathies produced by continued gouty pain, and which are erroneously ascribed to gouty *repulsion*, but which in fact are solely attributable to gouty *station*.

The perseverance with which the remedy in the instance related, was applied, was necessary to effectuating a cure, but it probably would have been shortened, if the slightest sensation of either originating or recurring pain in the different joints that were alternately attacked, had been repressed by topical cold. The painful degree of inflammatory heat would then most likely have not obtained, and the patient would have been exempted from afflicting relapses. The case seems peculiarly well adapted for general immersion. When a strong disposition to ligamentous and tendinous excitement exists, it indicates a distempered susceptibility in that structure for inflammatory affection, and is most effectually subdued by the refrigerant and tonic influence of general cold bathing. K.

z " Thus

" Thus accident produces to the ignorant sometimes a remedy without reason, and which is brought into practice founded on reason, with all its advantages *.

" Why should we despair that fevers may not be treated by immersion? Dr. Baynard, who wrote in the sixteenth century, insists on it, and proves it on himself; but it is thought at present so desperate a remedy, that it may yet for a time be deemed murder, though it is well known the savages of America treat a fever in this manner with success †. Wishing you every success in your laudable endeavour to enlighten mankind, for their own benefit,

                    " I remain,
" *Knowle House,*   " Sir, &c.
  May 18th, 1804.   " G. MONTAGU."

---

* This case affords decisive testimony in favour of the perfect safety, and infallible curative efficacy of reduced temperature in arthritic inflammation. It also evinces the untenable futility of imagining any danger to attend the relief of *pain*, in a disease in which *pain* constitutes both the whole immediate and future grievance.   K.

† The doctrine of morbid temperature is extensively and importantly applicable to the cure of diseases; and when social refinement and intellectual degeneracy shall have retraced their devious course to the instinctive rectitude of common sense, it will be as correctly as simply seen, and acknowledged, that water
                                                    extinguishes

Cases and Observations on gouty Affection, by Dr. Kinglake.

Two interesting cases of the happy success of topical cold, in speedily extinguishing gouty inflammation, have just reached me. One was an instance of chronic gout, affecting in turn, with inflammatory violence, all the joints of the lower extremities, with which also those of the upper limbs often painfully sympathized. ·

extinguishes fire by attenuating and distributing the concentrated force of repulsive motion, and that it operates in the same manner on both animate and inanimate matter. Until this auspicious æra shall arrive, the savages, or rather *sages* of America, will enjoy but too exclusively the salutary advantages of immersion in cold water during the hot stage of fever; a practice which the impulse of *natural feeling*, unbiassed by perverted *reason*, led them confidently to adopt. However abortive may be the attempt, it is my intention, with all convenient speed, to wield a spear in the service of humanity, against the *enchanted*, the *paradoxical* prejudice that contends for the propriety of attempting the reduction of heat by augmenting its force. My object is to found and arrange the theory and cure of diseases on the principle of temperature. It must be confessed that this design, in the present state of medical knowledge, cannot be satisfactorily accomplished; but this obstacle should not delay its commencement. Much immediate benefit will result from the research; it also opens a wide field for scientific emulation, in which the combined talents and industry of the medical faculty promise to be sufficiently exerted to ensure the inquiry at no very distant period its desirable completion. K.

The

The disease had existed during several months, and had been unavailingly treated in the usual manner. An inability either to rise from the bed, or to exert any degree of locomotion, resulted from its uninterrupted continuance and unmitigated severity. Under these circumstances, topically bathing the affected parts with cold water, at short intervals, afforded immediate relief to the pain; and, in the course of a few weeks, enabled the patient to be again on his feet, and daily to get on horseback.

The local feebleness necessarily arising from so long disuse of the affected ligaments and tendons still remains, but without any painful sense of morbid temperature.

This debility of the joints is also gradually lessening, and will no doubt, in due time, be superseded by the natural state of motive energy.

It is worthy of remark, that neither opiate nor sudorific medicine, given in large doses, made the least impression on the torture of the disease, nor had any thing afforded the smallest alleviation before the use of topical cold.

This.

This case furnishes an instance of that immeasurably lingering kind of gout, in which the most timid apprehension of established practice, respecting *repulsion*, is amply satisfied, in which sufficient time is supposed to have been allowed for the complete escape of all *material virus*, and in which an attempt to avert the impending decrepitude is judged vindicable. Agreeably to this reasoning, the patient had, on a former occasion, been subjected to the influence of the warm bath, and the usual stimulant applications to the affected parts, but without obtaining any sensible benefit. After several months discontinuance of all means of cure, and daily endeavouring to move the stiffened and painful limbs, the motive power was slowly restored, and the morbid irritation at length subsided.

It may be safely admitted as a practical maxim in the treatment of arthritic disease, whether of an acute or chronic description, that the pain invariably attending it, originates from morbid excess of heat; that the grievance, from its very nature, can only be appropriately and effectually subdued by its adequate reduction; and that the topical application of cold water, duly conducted, is a remedy as *infallible* as *simple*.

z 3

The

The other case is an example of the acute form of gouty inflammation, attacking with the usual violence the metacarpal joints. This was rapidly extinguished (as had been often previously effected) by immersing the diseased hand in cold water.

The patient, on former occasions, had been frequently harassed by sympathetic irritation on other joints, both before and after the removal of the primary paroxysm; to obviate which, he had recourse to the daily use of general cold bathing, with the desired effect of completely preventing all farther inconvenience.

The morbid sympathies liable to be generated in the ligamentous and tendinous structure throughout the whole frame, by acute gout, may no doubt be repressed and annihilated by the refrigerant and tonic influence of cold bathing. The redundant heat and motive agitation, pervading the system during the convalescent stage of gouty disease, promise, by yielding to the evaporant and strengthening virtue of general immersion in cold water, to limit the affection to the part originally attacked, and to prevent its sympathetically kindling into inflammatory excitement on other joints. Considerable experience

rience already warrants the opinion, that an early and persevering use of cold bathing in the period of recovery from gouty affection, will prove highly beneficial, both in a preventive and restorative view of its efficacy. With but few exceptions, the decline of morbid temperature, whether inflammatory or febrile, acute or chronic, may be expedited and confirmed by daily immerging in cold water. The remnant portion of preternatural temperature, which still sustains diseased excitement, is detached by its influence, and vital power is progressively recruited, until the salutary standard of heat and action is fully reinstated. The practice of attempting to strengthen the feeble system, during convalescence, by stimulant treatment, is surely repugnant to its object. The motive power of life is but just emerging from the exhausting violence of morbid excitement, every fibre is yet sore from the struggle, and tremulously alive to renewed commotion.

The conflict, which has been endured, arose from stimulant violence; and is it consistent with a rational attempt to further the retrieval of strength, to replunge the motive power of life, enfeebled and tottering almost to its downfal, into its late agitation? But is not this the

tendency,

tendency, and in fact often the effect, of endeavouring to accelerate convalescence, by prematurely resorting to a full diet, a liberal portion of wine, medicinal tonics, and social intercourse? These indulgences should be sparingly commenced, and only gradually extended, as radical amendment of strength may be able to endure, and appear to require additional succour.

The regeneration of lost energy, in vital power, is not a rapid process; its salutary course is governed by many precarious circumstances of distempered excitability; it must be exactly regulated by the existing condition of motive power. If the excitement induced by the means employed be disproportionate to the reactive power of life, an agitated and exhausting effect will be produced, instead of augmented and permanent strength.

The increased susceptibility of the system for undue impression from every stimulant cause, is so great in all cases of weakness, whether in connexion with the early or declining stage, of either acute or chronic affection, that the leading practical difficulty consists in avoiding noxious excitement. The nutritive support, which

which is indispensably necessary, is often pur-
chased at the serious price of temporarily aggravating the prevailing disorder. But á comparatively small quantity of alimentary sustenance is
requisite, even in health, to that which is commonly taken; and very little indeed is abundantly sufficient in reconducting the disordered
motion of vital power to a state of healthful
regularity.

Abstemious diet, aqueous dilution, an habitually low temperature, daily immersion in cold
water succeeded by brisk friction, and mental
tranquillity, are best adapted to nurse and mature
the nascent strength of gouty convalescence, in
common with that of most other diseases.

Taunton,   Robert Kinglake.
July 5th, 1804.

ADDRESS

MEDICAL FACULTY.

DR. KINGLAKE acknowledges his sincere obligation to those of his medical brethren, who have liberally furnished him with their experience, in support of the salutary efficacy of topical cold in gouty inflammation.

He farther entreats an occasional communication of their practical remarks on the subject. Dr. K. also again solicits both the medical profession and public at large, to transmit to him the occurrence of any additional testimony that may be thought conducive to the true interests of the remedy, and to the lasting benefit of mankind.

Dr. K. has no difficulty in averring his conviction of the validity of his theoretic and practical doctrine of gout to be as complete as any purpose of rational confidence could require.

When

When a similar persuasion shall pervade the medical world, the popular prejudice against it will subside, and gout will then take its legitimate station among the slightest and most easily curable diseases; instead of ranking, as at present, with the most virulent and intractable.

With a view to the early attainment of this desirable end, Dr. K. proposes to publish as often as he shall be enabled (he hopes at least annually) a faithful report of the refrigerant practice in gouty inflammation, whether obtained from the invited intelligence of correspondents, or from his own experience.

By this procedure, Dr. K. thinks it fair to presume, that in the course of a few years the subject will be fully illustrated and correctly appreciated.

" Homo naturæ minister et interpres tantum facit et intelligit quantum de ordine naturæ *opere* vel *mente* observaverit : nec amplius scit aut potest." BACON.

Taunton,
July 5th, 1804.

THE END.

The

The Two following original Works are preparing
for the Press, and speedily will be published, by
the Author of this Dissertation.

I.

THOUGHTS

ON

MEDICINAL OPERATION;

OR,

A philosophical Inquiry into the various Modes in which salutary
Influence is exerted, in alleviating and curing Diseases.

II.

THERMONOSOLOGIA;

OR,

THE DOCTRINE OF MORBID TEMPERATURE.

Exhibiting a View of the Nature, Prevention, and Cure of the
diseased Effects of excessive and deficient Heat in the Animal
Economy;

WITH

A CRITICAL INQUIRY

Into the Use and Abuse of the prevailing Practice of Medicine.

Also a Translation, by the same Author, from the original
German, of Professor TROMSDORFF's

CHEMICAL ART OF PRESCRIBING;

INTENDED AS

A VADE MECUM

FOR

MEDICAL PRACTITIONERS,

Who, in extemporaneously ordering Medicine, would avoid
chemical and pharmaceutical Errors.

With extensive Additions by the Translator, by which the
Work is more usefully adapted to British Practitioners of
Medicine.

4   A LIST

A LIST OF

MEDICAL BOOKS,

AND

ANATOMICAL PLATES,

Published since March 1802,

BY JOHN MURRAY, MEDICAL BOOKSELLER, LONDON.

ANATOMICAL PLATES.

1. JOHN GOTTLIEB WALTER's PLATES of the THORACIC and ABDOMINAL NERVES, reduced from the Original, as published by Order of the Royal Academy of Sciences at Berlin: accompanied by coloured Explanations, and a Description of the PAR VAGUM, GREAT SYMPATHETIC and PHRENIC NERVES. Elegantly printed in large 4to. price 18s. in boards.

" Professor Walter's incomparable plates are well known by anatomists to be one of the most accurate, most complete, and altogether most perfect specimens of neurology ever published ; they are executed in the most masterly style of engraving. Being not easily procurable, Dr. Hooper has done a great service to anatomy in republishing them in a reduced form, accompanied with the original explanations, to which he has added a short account of the par vagum, and great sympathetic and phrenic nerves. Dr. H. has also adopted the very useful plan of some of his former anatomical selections, of accompanying the finished plate with a variously coloured outline skeleton, to which all letters of reference are transferred ; a plan which preserves the unity and clearness of the engraving, and is of the most material assistance to the reader. The plates of this collection are executed in a remarkably distinct and elegant manner, and do great credit to the artist, Mr. Kirtland."—*Aikin's Annual Review,* vol. ii. p. 772.

" The merit of the original author of these plates deserves every commendation. The situation of the nerves described in the human body, their organs, plexuses, ganglia, and other connexions, are pointed out with a minuteness and accuracy hitherto unequalled. The extreme intricacy and difficulty of the subject heighten the merit of the execution ; and when we consider the importance of the particular nerves here treated of, to the human constitution, we shall feel ourselves called upon to acknowledge with gratitude the utility of his labours.—The reduced copy, which is here presented to us, deserves praise for the fidelity and clearness with which it is executed. The par vagum, the great sympathetic nerve, and the phrenic nerve, not having been described by Walter, a description of them is added in the present work; and it is but justice to say, that, for precision and perspicuity, this addition does no discredit

discredit to the descriptions which it accompanies."—*Literary Journal for February* 16, 1804, p. 146.

2. A PLATE, engraved from a very accurate Drawing by KIRTLAND, exhibiting, at one View, the BLOOD-VESSELS of the HEAD, with their NAMES and REFERENCES. Price 7s. coloured.

3. A large folio PLATE, coloured, exhibiting the interior BLOOD-VESSELS of the ARM, price 10s. 6d.

4. An enlarged coloured VIEW of the EXTERNAL and INTERNAL EAR, from a Preparation of an eminent Surgeon, price 5s.

" From this plate the operation of puncturing the tympanum may be seen with great correctness."—*Aikin's Annual Review*, vol. ii. p. 766.

5. A single coloured PLATE, giving a very accurate transverse SECTION of the EYE, much magnified, accompanied with a short EXPLANATION. By Dr. HOOPER, price 3s.

" The length of the figure is nine inches, which is well adapted for demonstration in a lecture-room."—*Aikin's Annual Review*, vol. ii. p. 766.

" Where actual inspection of the parts cannot be obtained, these faithful delineations are of great and undoubted utility; and they may be studied with advantage by all, but more particularly by the junior part of the profession."—*Medical and Chirurgical Review*, vol. xi. p. 62.

6. ANATOMICAL PLATES of the BONES and MUSCLES, diminished from ALBINUS; accompanied by EXPLANATORY MAPS. For the Use of Students. The second Edition, price 7s.

7. ANATOMICAL PLATES of the THORACIC and ABDOMINAL VISCERA; accompanied by EXPLANATORY MAPS. For the Use of Students, price 5s.

" The figures in these two little volumes are very neatly and very accurately executed, and are accompanied by maps, or separate outlines, differently coloured, which render the explanation and reference very easy. The whole forms a very neat, portable, and useful help to the student."—See *Physical Journal*, vol. viii. p. 473; and *Aikin's Annual Review*, vol. i. p. 849, &c.

———————

The ANATOMIST'S VADE-MECUM, containing the ANATOMY, PHYSIOLOGY, MORBID APPEARANCES, &c. of the HUMAN BODY, the ART of making ANATOMICAL PREPARATIONS, &c. The FIFTH Edition, considerably enlarged. To which are now
added,

added, ANATOMICAL, PHYSIOLOGICAL, MEDICAL, and SURGI-
CAL QUESTIONS for STUDENTS. By ROBERT HOOPER, M. D.
Fellow of the Linnæan and London Medical Societies, Resident
Physician to the St. Mary-le-bonne Infirmary, &c. &c.—In one
very closely printed volume, small octavo, price 9s. in boards.

The above Work presents to the Student a useful Anatomical
Conspectus, or Pocket Manual of Anatomy and Physiology: in
which he will find, 1. A short but accurate Description of the
different Parts of the Human Body, and their Functions.—2. An
Enumeration of the Diseases to which those Parts are subject,
and the various Operations of Surgery that are performed on the
Human Body.—3. The Method of preparing the various Parts of
the Body, to exhibit their Structure in a healthy and diseased
State, as far as our present Knowledge will enable us.—4. A
Glossary, or Explanation of the principal Terms used in that
Science.—5. Such Questions as the Student will probably be required to answer at the College of Surgeons, the Medical Board,
the Board of Sick and Hurt, &c. in order to obtain his Diploma,
or pass as Surgeon or Surgeon's Mate for the Army or Navy, or
the Service of the East India Company.

" The utility of this performance in the English language, as well as
the manner in which it is executed, induce us to recommend it to all
students in anatomy and surgery."—*Medical and Physical Journal for March*
1800.

" The rapid sale of this compendium of anatomy is, in this instance, a
merited testimony to its value, and we only here notice the *fifth edition,*
to mention the anatomical questions, which make a small accession to the
volume ; they are one hundred and forty-eight in number, and sufficiently
well chosen."—*Physical Journal,* 1804, vol. xi. p. 189.

The LONDON DISSECTOR ; or a COMPENDIUM of PRACTICAL
ANATOMY: containing a DESCRIPTION of the MUSCLES, VES-
SELS, NERVES, and VISCERA of the HUMAN BODY, as they ap-
pear on DISSECTION ; with DIRECTIONS for their DEMONSTRA-
TION. 12mo. boards, 5s.

" This will be found a very useful guide to the student in the prosecution of his anatomical researches. It is superior to other works of a
similar kind and extent, in describing not the muscles merely, but the
various parts, blood-vessels, nerves, &c. as they come into view under
the knife of the dissector. A knowledge of the relative situation of parts
is thus acquired, a point of the first magnitude to the practical surgeon.
As the chief intention of the work is to teach the art of dissecting, the
muscles are demonstrated in their order of situation, which is the only
method that can be pursued in actual dissection."—*Medical and Chirurgical
Review,* 1804, vol. xi. p. 62.

A short DESCRIPTION of the HUMAN MUSCLES, arranged as
they appear on Dissection ; together with their several Uses, and
the

the Synonyma of the best Authors. By John Innes. A new Edition, with considerable Alterations and Improvements: illustrated with Sixteen Plates, descriptive of the Bones and Muscles. 12mo. price 7s. 6d. in boards.

The Elements of Physiology, containing a comprehensive View and clear Explanation of the Functions of the Human Body, in which the modern Improvements in Chemistry, Galvanism, and other Sciences are applied, to explain the Actions of the Animal Economy; with a new Classification, and a copious Index. Translated from the French of A. Richerand, Professor of Anatomy and Physiology, and principal Surgeon of the Hospital of the North, in Paris, by Robert Kerrison, Member of the Royal College of Surgeons in London, &c. In one closely printed volume, 8vo. price 9s. in boards.

" This work is upon the whole very well executed, full of the necessary information, and not abounding with frivolous or irrelevant matter; so that the author must both have had very good teachers, and must have profited largely from the advantages of education."—*Medical and Physical Journal*, vol. x. p. 568.

" Various treatises and observations on different parts of the animal economy, have recently been published by Bordieu, Richart, Barthez, Hall, Fourcroy, &c. To these sources, and particularly to the manuscript Lectures of Grimand, the author of the present work acknowledges himself to be greatly indebted, as well as to the works of Haller and Sœmmering. The facts derived from all these authorities, as well as from his own observations, he has arranged with considerable ingenuity, and brought under one point of view in the present compendium. The translator appears to have executed his task with fidelity."—*British Critic for Dec.* 1803, p. 610.

" This work will be found useful to those who are desirous of becoming acquainted with some of the general doctrines of physiology, and it may serve as a work of reference to those who may want to refresh their memory with the rudiments of this science."—*Aikin's Annual Review*, vol. ii. p. 758.

The Lectures of the celebrated Boyer upon the Diseases of the Bones, arranged into a systematic Treatise, by A. Richerand, Professor of Anatomy and Physiology, and principal Surgeon to the Northern Hospital at Paris. Translated from the French, by M. Farrell, M.D. In 2 vols. 8vo. price 14s. in boards.

*** The work of Boyer contains some important discoveries relative to the diseases upon which it treats, and points out many new and successful modes of treatment, which have been sanctioned and adopted by the most eminent practitioners upon the continent.

ILLUS-

ILLUSTRATIONS of some of the INJURIES to which the lower LIMBS are exposed, accompanied by COLOURED PLATES. By CHARLES BRANDON TRYE, Member of the late Corporation of Surgeons, in London, of the Royal Medical Society in Edinburgh, and Surgeon to the Gloucester Infirmary. 4to. 6s. 6d.

" Observations of this kind, made from cases actually occurring, are always valuable. The author has had the opportunity of examining, in two instances, after death, the state of parts deranged by violent, but not of itself fatal, external injury, &c. These cases are the basis of the present work, and have furnished seven plates of the appearances after dissection."—*Aikin's Annual Review*, vol. ii. p. 775.

" The subjects here illustrated are, dislocations of the thigh bone, fractures of the neck of the thigh bone, dislocation of the astragalus, deformity of the knees and legs in children, and the club-foot. The cases of dislocation and fracture are well described, and the observations throughout are pertinent and judicious."—*British Critic*.

A DISSERTATION on GOUT; exhibiting a new View of the Origin, Nature, Cause, Cure, and Prevention of that afflicting Disease, illustrated and confirmed by a Variety of original and communicated Cases. By ROBERT KINGLAKE, M.D. Member of the Royal Medical Society of Edinburgh; of the Physical Society of Gottingen, &c. &c. and Physician at Taunton. 8vo. price 7s. 6d.

A concise and systematic ACCOUNT of a painful AFFECTION of the NERVES of the FACE, commonly called TIC DOULOUREUX. By S. FOTHERGILL, M.D. Physician to the Western Dispensary. 8vo. price 3s. sewed.

OUTLINES of a TREATISE on the DISORDERED STATE of the LUNGS; intended to illustrate the ORIGIN and NATURE of many of the most IMPORTANT DISEASES; and also to afford proper Indications to assist in their Treatment and Prevention. 8vo. price 5s.

" The anonymous author of this pamphlet is of the eccentric kind. He appears to be not unversed in medical reading ; and there are some pertinent and even original observations interspersed in this book."— *British Critic*, May 1804, p. 557.

OBSERVATIONS on the EPIDEMICAL DISEASES now prevailing in London; with their Divisions, Method of Treatment, Prevention, &c. By ROBERT HOOPER, M.D. Resident Physician to the St. Mary-le-bonne Infirmary, &c. 8vo. price 1s. 6d.

" This very interesting treatise we earnestly recommend to all our readers, as containing much important information concerning the epidemic which has been so generally prevalent in this metropolis. The matter of fact contained in this treatise is highly valuable, and the practice laid down is judicious and discriminative."—*Medical Journal*, vol. ix. p. 387.

A CON-

A CONSPECTUS of the LONDON and EDINBURGH PHARMACO-POEIAS; wherein the Virtues, Uses, and Doses of the several Articles and Preparations contained in these Works, are concisely stated; their Pronunciation, as to Quantity, is correctly marked, and a Variety of other Particulars respecting them given, calculated more especially for the Use of junior Practitioners. By ROBERT GRAVES, M.D. F.L.S. Member of the Royal College of Physicians, London, &c. Third Edition, corrected, and adapted to the last improved Editions of the Colleges. Price 3s. 6d. sewed.

MEDICAL SKETCHES of the EXPEDITION to EGYPT from INDIA. By JAMES M'GREGOR, A.M. Member of the Royal College of Surgeons of London, Surgeon to the Royal Horse Guards, and lately Superintending Surgeon of the Indian Army in Egypt. In 8vo. price 7s. boards.

" The object of the author appears to have been, to lay before the world a clear and correct statement of facts, which may be of the last import-ance to those who devote themselves to the investigation of the particular diseases which are here described. Considering the work in this point of view, we have no hesitation in saying, that this is a very useful publica-tion, and well worthy the serious attention of the medical body, particu-larly of those gentlemen who may be called upon to practise in the East and West Indies, or any hot climate."—*Literary Journal.*

" Mr. M'G. appears to be a diligent observer and an accurate reporter of what he has seen, with little bias to doubtful speculations, or hypo-theses. His work, therefore, will be read with considerable interest, and will hereafter furnish some valuable documents for illustrating the me-dical history of Egypt, and of inter-tropical climates in general."—*Medical and Chirurgical Review for July* 1804, p. 35.

OBSERVATIONS on DIARRHOEA and DYSENTERY, as those Diseases appeared in the BRITISH ARMY, during the Campaign in EGYPT, in 1801. To which are prefixed, a Description of the Climate of Egypt, and a Sketch of the Medical History of the Campaign. By HENRY DEWAR, late Assistant Surgeon to the 30th, or Cambridgeshire Regiment of Foot. 8vo. price 4s. boards.

" This description of dysentery is drawn up with great clearness, good sense, and accuracy; and, on the whole, we may consider this treatise as another instance of the excellent field of observation even the military hospital furnishes, to those who have been rendered adequate to it by previous study."—*Medical Journal,* vol. x. p. 282-3.

" Mr. Dewar has published some interesting observations on diarrhoea and dysentery, &c. They evince a considerable share of medical know-ledge, sound judgment, and accurate remark."—*Monthly Magazine for June* 1804, p. 625.

An ATTEMPT to investigate the CAUSE of the EGYPTIAN OPHTHALMIA, with Observations on the Nature and different

Modes

Modes of Cure. By GEORGE POWER, Assistant Surgeon to the 23d Regiment of Foot, or Royal Welch Fusileers. 8vo. price 2s. 6d.

" The author of this Essay had an opportunity, by being attached to the English army in Egypt, of seeing very numerous instances of the Egyptian ophthalmia, a disease which is peculiarly serious and obstinate. To this field of extensive observation, which enabled him to become acquainted with every form of the complaint, was added a severe attack of it in his own person, which gave him occasion to try the effects of opium, which he did with so much success, that from that time it formed a part of the plan of the military hospital appropriated to ophthalmic patients; and it is affirmed as a fact, that, in the space of a month from its general use, every one of them was restored to the army, in a state either of convalescence or of perfect health."—*Aikin's Annual Review,* vol. ii. p. 731.

" We have been highly gratified with the perusal of this sensible and well-written pamphlet. The author was attached to the medical staff of the British army that served during the campaign in Egypt in 1801, and had the charge of several hundred patients afflicted with complaints incidental to the climate.

" We forbear to conduct our readers through the remaining chapters of this interesting performance, which contain a full description of the several varieties and progressive stages of the disease in question; judicious comments on the practice of the native and European surgeons; and the account of a more successful method of treatment pursued under the author's direction in the hospital at Gheza."—*Imperial Review for April* 1803, p. 587, &c.

A TREATISE on CHELTENHAM WATERS and BILIOUS DISEASES; containing, 1. The chemical and medical Properties of the saline Springs of Cheltenham and its Neighbourhood.—2. Arrangement and History of Bilious Diseases occurring in this Country.—3. The Uses of the saline Waters in curing Diseases.—4. Directions for the most appropriate Mode of drinking the Waters.—5. Geological Experiment for the Discovery of new saline Springs at Cheltenham.—6. The Nature and Uses of the Steel Well, in Mr. Barrett's Field. To which are prefixed, Observations on Fluidity, Mineral Waters, and Watering Places. By THOMAS JAMESON, M. D. Member of the College of Physicians of London and Edinburgh, &c. &c. In octavo, price 6s. in boards.

" This volume will be of great use to the invalid who visits Cheltenham on account of his health."—*European Magazine for April* 1804, p. 295.

An INQUIRY into the LAWS of CHEMICAL AFFINITY. By C. L. BERTHOLLET, Member of the Conservative Senate and National Institution. Translated from the French by M. FARRELL, M. D. In 8vo. price 7s. in boards.

A TREATISE,

A TREATISE, shewing the INTIMATE CONNEXION that subsists between AGRICULTURE and CHEMISTRY, addressed to the Cultivators of the Soil; to the Proprietors of Fens and Peat Mosses in Great Britain and Ireland; and to the Proprietors of West India Estates. By the Earl of DUNDONALD. A new Edition, 1 vol. 4to. price 10s. 6d. in boards.

The novelty and importance of this design, and the genius and felicity with which it has been executed by the Noble Author, are admitted by the best judges of chemistry, and particularly by men highly distinguished for the application of philosophy to mechanical and practical pursuits. To give a list of such names as Dr. Pearson, the Bishop of Landaff, &c. &c. in support of this assertion, might be thought improper. The publishers, therefore, refer the public, for the character of this work, to the following periodical publications, which profess to estimate literary and scientific merit; for although the testimony of any one of these might be deemed equivocal, their universal concurrence in the highest commendations of the Earl of Dundonald's Treatise on Chemical Agriculture, cannot but have weight with every mind.

The Gentleman's Magazine for April 1795, p. 323.
The European Magazine for May 1795, p. 320.
The Analytical Review for July 1795.
The English Review for May and June 1795.
The Critical Review for June 1795.
The Monthly Review for September 1795.

ELEMENTS of SCIENCE and ART; being a familiar INTRODUCTION to NATURAL PHILOSOPHY and CHEMISTRY. Together with their Application to a Variety of elegant and useful Arts. By JOHN IMISON. A new Edition, considerably enlarged, and adapted to the improved State of Science. Illustrated by Thirty Plates, by LOWRY. Two Volumes, 8vo. price 1l. 5s.

" John Imison, the original author of this improved work, was an ingenious and industrious mechanic. His original publication was considered as affording so much practical information, that it became conspicuously distinguished among books of this class, and passed through not less than eight editions.

" The very extensive improvement in all branches of natural philosophy, which of late years has taken place, rendered various additions and alterations indispensably necessary to a new edition of Imison's work. This task has been undertaken, and these additions supplied, by Mr. Webster, who was assistant to the late Dr. Garnett, at the Royal Institution.

" The plates, which are thirty-two in number, are executed with remarkable neatness and perspicuity by Lowry, who has before distinguished himself by his ingenuity in this line. The book is also exceedingly well printed; and the whole may very properly be recommended to students in natural philosophy, as a convenient and not expensive manual."—*British Critic, March* 1804, p. 252.

ELEMENTS of GALVANISM, in THEORY and PRACTICE; with a comprehensive VIEW of its HISTORY from the FIRST EXPERIMENTS

of

of GALVANI to the PRESENT TIME. Containing also, Practical Directions for constructing the Galvanic Apparatus, and plain systematic Instructions for performing all the various Experiments. By C. H. WILKINSON, S. A. S. Lecturer on Galvanism in Soho Square, Member of the Royal College of Surgeons, of the Philosophical Society of Manchester, &c. &c. 2 vols. 8vo. illustrated with a great Number of Copper-plates, price 1l. 1s. in boards.

" The reader will find interwoven with the first principles and fundamental experiments of Galvanism, a considerable body of useful information, related in a pleasing manner, without ostentation, and yet free from any thing low and mean.

" In PARALYTIC AFFECTIONS, Galvanism has often proved of very considerable advantage.

" In cases of DEAFNESS considerable relief has been afforded by means of Galvanism.

" With regard to the influence of Galvanism in cases of MENTAL DERANGEMENT, Mr. W. mentions its good effect in two instances, by Aldini.

" In NERVOUS HEADACHES, to which females are subject, accompanied by violent oppressive sensation over the eyes, with an almost entire inability of motion, Galvanism is of the greatest advantage, &c.

" The discoveries in the science of Galvanism have, during the last few years, excited the attention of almost every person engaged in the pursuit of natural and experimental philosophy during the last twelve years, or has excited an almost universal attention.—The progress it has made has been exceedingly rapid.

" It is now fourteen years since Galvani, the celebrated Italian from whom the science derives its name, was accidentally led to a series of experiments, which have been succeeded by others, than which, perhaps, none more brilliant and astonishing were ever exhibited to the world."— *Imperial Review, April* 1804, p. 554, &c.

" The discovery of Galvanism has laid open a field of inquiry, at once so novel, so important, and so diversified, that no one can wonder at the eagerness and curiosity with which it is still pursued.

" This work may be considered as presenting an accumulation of valuable facts relative to the promulgation, establishment, progress, and present state of Galvanism, and as holding forth a reasonable expectation of the most important advantages to be derived from its further cultivation."—*European Mag. Jan.* 1804, p. 40.

" In two octavo volumes, illustrated with many curious plates, the learned lecturer illustrates the doctrine of Galvanism in a scientific but clear detail, which we recommend to the perusal of our readers."— *Gentleman's Mag. May* 1804, p. 447.

" The author of this production has performed an acceptable service to the public, by collecting and arranging the various facts and doctrines which have appeared in different quarters on the subject of Galvanism, and thus afforded a corrected view of the progress and present state of this science.

" Thirteen well-executed plates illustrate this publication, and it is judiciously furnished with an ample index."—*Monthly Review, Jan.* 1804, p. 201.

LEPI-

LEPIDOPTERA BRITANNICA; containing the Latin and English Names, a NEW ARRANGEMENT and NEW DESCRIPTION of Seventy-two Species of PAPILIO; Twenty-eight SPHINGES; Four ZYGÆNÆ; and Ninety-eight BOMBYCES; with all the Synonyms, Food, Times and Places of Appearance in their different States, and Measure of their Wings: also an Account of all their Peculiarities, and the best Modes of destroying such as are injurious to Mankind. To which are added, Six Botanical Dissertations, viz. A new Arrangement and Descriptions of Two Hundred and Eleven Species of Mesembryanthemum—A new Arrangement of the Genus Tetragonia—A new Arrangement of the Genus Portulacca —A new Arrangement of the Genus Saxifraga—A Dissertation on Twenty-four new Species of exotic Plants—And a Dissertation on the Technical Terms of the Science of Botany. By A. H. HAWORTH, F. L. S. 8vo. price 15s. in boards.

" The plan on which the present work is constructed, is different from any other that has been adopted, and is remarkable for precision and distinctness. The work is besides recommended by the novelty of its sectional, generic, and specific characters; the amplitude of the general descriptions, of which the merit and invention belong almost solely to the author, and the novelty and excellence of the observations, which occasionally follow these descriptions. The author has also given a description of the time of feeding, the food, the times of the flight, and the measure of the wings, which is equally novel, entertaining, and instructive. His diligence was such, that,. with few exceptions, he has seen the different species here described in a living state. But the work is not only valuable to the man of science, by the perspicuity and precision of the technical descriptions, but must prove highly entertaining and instructive even to the general reader, on account of the curious and interesting observations, which frequently occur. The work, both as to its plan and its execution, can scarcely be too highly praised, and is beyond comparison the best publication which has hitherto appeared on the British Lepidoptera."—*Literary Journal, May* 1, 1804, p. 473, &c.

The SOLDIER'S FRIEND; containing Familiar Instructions to the Loyal Volunteers, Yeomanry Corps, and Military Men in general, on the Preservation and Recovery of their Health; arranged under the following Heads: Preliminary Remarks; Wounds and other Casualties; Camps and Barracks; Cleanliness; Exercise; Military Dress; Weather; Diet and Cookery; Intemperance; Prevention of Disease; Hospitals and Nursing; Appendix and Additions; with a prefatory Address to Commanding Officers. By W. BLAIR, A. M. Member of the Royal College of Surgeons; Fellow of the Medical Societies of London, Paris, and Brussels; Surgeon of the Lock Hospital and Asylum, and of the Bloomsbury Dispensary, &c. In a neat Pocket Volume (being a new Edition, considerably enlarged, and illustrated by Eight Engravings), price 5s. in boards.

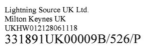

Lightning Source UK Ltd.
Milton Keynes UK
UKHW012128061118
331891UK00009B/526/P

9 780483 581050